# GOODBYE TO CLOCKS TICKING

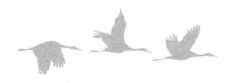

*How We Live While Dying*

— A MEMOIR —

JOSEPH MONNINGER

STEERFORTH PRESS
LEBANON, NEW HAMPSHIRE

For information about permission to reproduce
selections from this book, write to:
Steerforth Press L.L.C., 31 Hanover Street, Suite 1,
Lebanon, New Hampshire 03766

Cataloging-in-Publication Data is available from the Library of Congress

ISBN 978-1-58642-360-5 (Hardcover)

Manufactured in the United States of America

1 3 5 7 9 10 8 6 4 2

*This book is dedicated to my fellow cancer patients.
I see you and I know you see me.*

*Live your life, do your work, then take your hat.*

— HENRY DAVID THOREAU

# 1

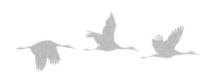

I'm dying.

We're all dying, of course. Everyone who is born begins to die the moment after they gulp air and cry out. Talking about dying is an intellectually safe game to play. We can talk about death, about how we would behave in this or that crisis, and then we can spin confidently back to whatever we were doing a moment before and reassure ourselves that we are not there yet.

Not ready to die. Too young. Too strong. Not our turn.

My train — a hackneyed cliché, but it *is* a train, because if we listen we can hear it coming toward us — arrived on an afternoon in May 2021, three days after I retired.

Three days.

That's not a joke or a typo. After thirty-two years of teaching college classes, after a ballpark guess of working with six thousand students, after planning for my modest savings to be shepherded correctly, after signing up for Social Security and Medicare, I visited my primary physician to say I had been experiencing shortness of breath for a few weeks. The primary physician put a stethoscope to my back, listened, moved it once or twice, listened some more, and then said, "Let's get you an X-ray."

The X-ray, it turns out, was *concerning*. The doctor recommended I have a CT scan of my lungs just to make sure nothing strange was afoot. I went to Speare Memorial Hospital in

Plymouth, New Hampshire, and had a CT scan, after which the young radiology technician asked if I'd ever had surgery on my lungs.

"No," I answered, "but now you have me concerned."

"Oh, it's nothing," she hurried to reassure me. "It could be anything."

The train came a little closer.

In 2019, I purchased a small cottage in Pembroke, Maine. It was a retired post office, a creaky old building dragged to the site by a former local high school teacher who sold biological materials to commercial school markets. He intended to run a kayaking business out of it, or turn it into a playhouse for his kids. The building was in rough shape, thirteen by twenty feet, but it was approximately fifty yards away from Pennamaquan Bay, a beautiful river estuary that feeds into Cobscook Bay and from there to the Bay of Fundy. The building gave me more pleasure than I had anticipated. It came with two good acres sloping toward the bay. No running water or electricity. No heat except for a coal stove. In the online world, in the world of Covid, the cottage seemed a refuge. My life partner, Susan, loved the place as much as I did, and we spent lovely days sitting in the sun on the front deck or hiking to Quoddy Head Point, or watching the lobster boats ply the waters off Roque Bluffs Beach. It was, we promised each other, a place to retire. We walked the grounds and decided where a simple home could go. Given the proximity to the bay, we found it was easy to have a 180-degree view of the water. The old post office could serve as a guest cottage. The plans — the idea of building something, the possibility that I might contribute as a retired man to the carpentry — filled my days with dreams. I watched videos about homesteading, researched outhouses and water cisterns. This was the future I had planned for many years during my working life. Now I had made it. No more school for me. No more classes or expectant faces raised to me to ask a question about the material.

All of that was behind me. Hammer and nails from now on. Carpentry.

I had a shovel in my hand when the call came in from a different radiologist saying she had read my CT scan.

"Can you get back Monday?" she asked.

"I'm seven hours away. Can you tell me what's going on?"

She put me on hold. I realized later that she was weighing the ethics and legal peril of telling me such compromising information over the phone. She came back on a moment later, apologized for the delay, then with a resolved voice informed me that my chest scan had been "concerning" and that I had lung cancer. My primary doctor wanted to see me. I needed to go back to my home in New Hampshire.

"I'm up here on a fishing trip," I said, which was true. "We're going out for salmon."

"Well," she said.

I hung up a few minutes later after making plans to return the following week. Susan was due in an hour. I used the shovel to move some dirt around on the soggy, springtime driveway. Lung cancer. I had lung cancer. Up until that point, at sixty-seven, I took no medications, did not smoke or drink to excess. I hiked frequently around New Hampshire, and I usually took a daily walk of at least a half hour. I had monitored my eating as I approached retirement, and now I was twenty pounds lighter, with more maneuverability and energy. I felt good. No, I felt astonishingly good, ready to take on retirement and have fun. Months before my official retirement date, my email filled up with wishes for a happy retirement, for trips to be planned, for building designs.

In less than a week, it was all scotched. The dream of retirement, of ease and tranquillity, had disappeared in a single phone call.

*This is you*, the call reminded me, *not someone else.*

And as an old English teacher, I couldn't help asking—as e. e. cummings had asked about Buffalo Bill—*How do you like your blue-eyed boy, Mr. Death?*

*We all know we are dying, but nobody believes it.*

I had read that line somewhere in the past, but whether it is an accurate quote I can't determine. It's close enough. Oddly, one of the first thoughts I had after speaking to the radiologist was of "Her First Ball," a short story by the New Zealand writer Katherine Mansfield. I had taught the story many times but had only come to understand it fully in the past half decade. On its face, the story is simple. A young woman is going to her first ball. She is attending the soiree with her more worldly city cousins, and she can barely contain her excitement. The gaslights — the story was published in 1921, although it feels set in the 1890s — quiver with companionable joy. Everything around her intoxicates. She revels at the wonderful slipperiness of the dance floor, at the casual indifference of the men across the hall, at the solid pleasure her female cousins have in depending on their attentive brother. She dances with a partner, glides, swirls, catches her breath, dances again, is in love with the world, the light, the glittering movement. She has never felt so deliriously happy. Then, unexpectedly, an older gentleman appears to claim his dance from her tiny dance card. He is in his forties, still single, an attendee of too many social events. He is a veteran of the world, and of these lovely balls, and while he dances with her, capably but without any romance, he suggests that she will soon be one of the old ladies sitting on the stage to watch the youngsters, that the slippery floor will come to be a treacherous pond of bad footing, that she will be eager soon to have the dance finished so that she can return to her quiet bed.

You could argue he is death inserting himself into the fantasies of a young woman; for me, he is her mortality, the knowledge we have of our own ending while, simultaneously, denying it. We must dance with the older man, we must listen to him undermine our pleasant revel, but, equally important, we must forget him and cast him aside when he is finished poaching from our lives. That's what our young protagonist accomplishes. Her first ball is soured by the older man, and she is disconsolate, but then a younger, handsomer man comes to claim his dance, and in his arms the floor again becomes a miracle of gliding, the lights animated friends, the music divine. She bumps into the older man a few moments later and fails even to recognize him.

A story. That's all. I wondered why this story had come to mind, but then, just as quickly, I understood. This time, in my predicament, the older gentleman could not be so easily dismissed. This time there would be no continuing dance, no sublimation into a joyful present. The old man remained on the dance card, asking each time the music stopped if I was ready to go again, ready to climb up on the stage with the other old folks and begin counting the minutes until death released us. *We all know that we are dying, but nobody believes it.*

An hour after I had received the news about my bad CT scan, Susan arrived. She had known about the testing, of course, and had deliberately hurried her arrival so that she would be beside me when I received the news. Deep down, she had suspected the worst; so had I. But when she arrived, pulling down the grassy path to the old post office, she was nothing but smiles. Part of her happiness came from seeing me, I hoped, but the other part

— the larger part in that moment — was her arrival at the cottage. This building, this land, was our shared dream. Imagine, if you will, a small, shake-sided building with nine enormous windows, brown-roofed, with good, uncompromising lines, a front deck, and, behind it, a view of nothing but water. We were not rich people compared with many others — we have been teachers for most of our lives — and the cottage, sitting where it did, always felt as if we had won something for which we could never have hoped: a house on a hill, with clean sheets on the bed, lupines, harbor seals just off our property, scallop draggers anchored off the shore. Across the bay, Coggins Head was conservation land that would never be developed. Somehow, in this hasty world, we had found our way to this beautiful property, to a place that had arguably the finest night skies on the eastern seacoast. The moon rose out of the water to our east and slid along the neighboring shoreline chasing its reflection.

She rode in and our eyes met and we experienced nothing but happiness. In this mix, in this hollow exhalation of news that had altered my life so dramatically, we looked at each other and smiled, our joy at being back together in this place, our place, enough for the moment, enough for many days.

# 2

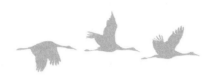

At our start, I saw Susan before she saw me.

She does not dispute the claim, but neither can she confirm it. I recall seeing her on a staircase in Rounds Hall, a stately four-story building on our Plymouth State campus, when she was a flight and a half above me. I looked up, and there she was. My memory contends that our eyes met for an instant, but my recounting of that moment is undermined by Susan's inability to recall me at all. In any case, I didn't know who she was or what she did on campus. It was only later, when we truly met, that I remembered she had appeared like a vision floating above me.

Perhaps I want the memory of our meeting to be more dramatic than it was, but when we finally did meet — on a faculty search committee to fill a slot in the English Department, where I was housed as a professor — we instantly liked each other. We sat across a table from each other while two colleagues, both serious and both intent on getting the right candidate for the job, devoured applications that Susan and I had taken less seriously. The incoming candidate was slated to work beside our two colleagues, so their stake in the search was far greater than ours. For Susan and me, serving on the committee was a form of university "service," an important third prong (in addition to scholarship and teaching) of our required commitment to the university's promotion and tenure calculations. We understood we were like outriggers on a canoe; we were there to make sure the search functioned properly and didn't swamp anyone in the process. University life is filled with these kinds of duties.

But we were attracted to each other. Later, after we had begun dating, Susan told me that she thought there was a space under my arm for her, a place to walk together.

Now, as she pulled in beside the post office, she smiled broadly. We both loved the house and land, and we both loved being there together. We did not live under the same roof; she was a mother of four young women, and I, well, I was a divorced man who was alone and who had a second career as a writer. We maintained separate residences so that she could be available to her girls and so that we could maintain a degree of independence. We liked leading our own lives, following our own interests, while also spending time together. The post office in Pembroke was our fortress and our favorite place to be. It was a house we shared.

She did not ask if I had heard from the doctor's office. It would have been unlike her to do so. Susan is as kind and as thoughtful as a human can be. At that moment beside the post office, she was fifty-five years old, a yogini, a lecturer for a Boston-based consortium on universal design for learning, a mom of four, a daughter to two aged parents, a sister in a family of five. Whenever I saw her after a small absence, I was reminded of the David Van Ronk song "Another Time and Place." The opening line of the song goes:

> *When first I met you years ago in another time and place*
> *The thought came to my mind that I had never seen a*
> *    kinder face.*

Yes, the kindest face I had ever seen. Soft, blue eyes and a warm, quiet presence that never failed to reassure me. We had both been through the absurd cattle-crossing of dating at older ages, and yet, somehow, we had managed to find each other. We knew we were lucky. That we could emerge as a couple, as people who found each other late in life, seemed an unlikely lottery win. Deep love, in other words. And great laughter.

We did the usual things to settle in, and we also followed our own rituals. We rang a marine bell — we rang three times when we arrived and departed — then spent a moment saying hello to a small cement statue of St. Francis. The St. Francis statue was a joke, but also an acknowledgment that we liked garden statuary. The bell and a hello to St. Francis. Then we grabbed her bags and moved her in.

How do you introduce the topic of severe illness? How do you insert into a conversation that you have had a word with your health provider, that there were *concerns*, that the young radiologist had asked about lung surgery, obviously having seen scars on the scan?

I found I couldn't broach the subject right away. But a little later on the deck as we watched the sunset, after we had established ourselves again in the post office, after we had eaten a lobster, after we had consumed two glasses of wine each, I tried to slide into our conversation that I had heard from the doctor's office.

Susan didn't ask what they had said. She simply reached over and held my hand.

"They said I have a mass in my left lung, and the cancer has metastasized into my liver and stomach and lymph nodes. And also into my brain," I said quietly. Then, to my surprise, I crumpled.

She slipped off her chair and came to kneel in front of me. We held each other. For the first time since I had heard from the radiologist's office, I realized I had at last spoken my fear aloud.

Discussing it, I became surprisingly choked up. I am not a particularly demonstrative man when it comes to the run of emotions, but I had little control over my feelings in those early conversations. Selfishly, my thinking continued to swirl around the central fact of my own position in the drama. It was not someone else; it was I who had this illness. Many times, I had received the news, as we all have, of a friend or colleague or even a family member having this or that diagnosis. It is difficult to hear, but then it passes quickly, relegated to those unfortunate things we hear about but can do nothing to resolve. But now, in this moment, I could not ignore the old man who had come to ask for a dance. My personal mortality was no longer theoretical. It had arrived at last in a stunning moment between my last day of work and my fourth day of retirement. The congestion I felt in my lung could no longer be explained away as a spot of hay fever. No, it was cancer, bad cancer, and my time had just been reduced from thoughts of a lovely, comfortable retirement to the possibility that I would not make it to Labor Day.

Susan and I slept close that night. We kept the screened door latched and uncovered to listen to the dawn chorus of gulls and songbirds. The sun lifted from Cobscook Bay, and the first rays spilled into our tiny home. *Now this has begun*, I remember thinking. *Now that I know I am dying.* Each breath became a measure weighed against my potential infirmity.

A new reality. Whereas before the phone call I had thought of the problem in my lung as being temporary, fixable, it now squatted inside my body with a solidness that I had not experienced before. The world had changed overnight. We were not going hiking now or ever after; we were not riding our bikes, one of our pleasures, to Pink Beach at the end of our road. Now a cough, even clearing my throat, became an indication of my illness. I was one thing the day before, quite another the day afterward.

We spent the morning in bed watching the sun establish itself in the east. The water in Pennamaquan Bay glistened. We had always loved to talk; it was one of our genuine pleasures. Under usual circumstances, our conversation roamed down ridiculous, whimsical side trails. We talked about education, about the risk of wearing bowling shoes, about the questionable taste of pineapples, and about the political future of our country. No subject usually held us for long, but now, in bed that first morning, we talked about my medical condition. Although we both understood we knew too little to draw intelligent conclusions, we couldn't resist theorizing about what the diagnosis meant. The conversation fed us; it allowed us to ward off the bigger, more dramatic questions — namely, How long did I have to live?

Most of life, I recognized, encouraged us to plot and plan. Susan and I were both highly verbal, and we had come this far by talking fast and negotiating with the world. Yet here, suddenly, was an argument too large, too one-sided to combat.

I had cancer. It was spreading. I knew, for the first time, how I would likely die.

"At least I won't die in a fire in Chicago," I said at some point that morning. "Most people don't know how they are going to die, but at least I have a pretty good idea how I will go."

"I always worry," Susan said, "that when something like this happens, and all the focus turns to one event, that something off the radar, something small but significant, will happen just out of our view. A friend will die in a car crash or something terrible will happen. I can't shake that feeling."

Later that morning my son, Justin, phoned to check in. The radiologist had called home the night before to get my cell number and he had given it out. We had talked, briefly, in the moments before Susan arrived. He had worked as an LNA at Dartmouth-Hitchcock, our state's biggest medical facility, and he had heard many diagnoses like the one I had received.

Most days we joked, but we didn't this morning. He asked how I felt. He asked what additional things the radiologist had said. I didn't know it then, but it would come to be a familiar conversational pattern. Well-intentioned friends and family members inquired after what news the last doctor had provided. The question, I realized eventually, had a variety of implications. While the interlocutor expressed concern and curiosity, the truth, I came to see, felt more complex. People asked questions because, somehow, they felt nothing was quite real until they had been given the chance to examine the full discourse. Perhaps they felt unconsciously that they would find some missing element in the news, or that they had to hear it themselves for it to be authentic, but the questions came at me consistently enough that I perceived it as a pattern.

And they also asked, I believed, because by knowing where death had traveled, they reassured themselves it was not at their door.

In any case, we chatted for a while. I told him what the weather was like, how the sun had come up, what we had planned for the day. He gave me his news. The year before he had returned from Thailand, where he had worked as a teacher, and he was now pursuing a similar position in the States. My news, he mentioned in passing, had made him withdraw his searches from faraway locations. He wanted to stay in New Hampshire; he wanted to help me through whatever it was I had to endure.

Susan drank coffee and painted a watercolor of Coggins Head. She had a goal to make a painting every time she visited the cottage. We listened to the gulls. This other thing, this broadside, undermined the slightest talk of the future. How do you plan for the future, even make tentative plans, when you didn't know what condition you would be in a fortnight from today?

I had another small problem: I had to inform my two fishing buddies, Bob and Ted, of my news. I considered holding out on them, letting them find me as they would, then telling them the full story when I possessed more solid information. But the truth was, the trip to fish Grand Lake Stream, a renowned salmon river, would require a level of physical fitness that I wasn't certain I could summon. Besides, we had been friends for a half century and had fished together every spring for more than forty years. We had been boys together, and it didn't seem fair to spring it on them.

I took my computer and drove to the Pembroke Town Hall, where I knew from experience I could get a Wi-Fi connection. I wrote them a quick note outlining what had transpired. I told them I wasn't ready to keel over, but I also needed them to know that something had changed. Truth was, we were approaching seventy and it was not a surprise, I supposed, that one of us could receive a diagnosis like this one. I confirmed that I still wanted our fishing trip to go forward. If the cancer proved deadly, as I imagined it would, then this could well be our last trip together.

I drove back to the post office, feeling — as I often would after the diagnosis— that this was all a bit of playacting. Everything in my life up until this point had been negotiable. I had escaped death at least three times, once at gunpoint in Wyoming; once in a well in Burkina Faso, West Africa; and once in the ocean off Point Pleasant, New Jersey. When I had first read in high school about Odysseus, I remember thinking that I understood his crafty intelligence, that it was, at least, a little like my own. I was not the smartest person in the room, nor the most disciplined, but when events demanded original solutions, thinking outside of the box, I usually fared pretty well. Driving beside the Pennamaquan River back to the post office, I was confident, absurdly as it turned out, that things would come right in the end. Yes, I had the news of my cancer, and yes, it appeared grave, but surely I could triumph in the end, skirt the clashing rocks or the swirling whirlpools and return to Ithaca at last.

Susan knew better. From the moment the diagnosis landed on us, she understood its full import. I was dying. The following day we had a phone call scheduled with a nurse practitioner to get more details. At the appointed time, we sat at the small table in our little post office and took the call. I put it on speaker so Susan could hear and ask questions of her own.

If we had expected relief, or a diminishment of the gravity of the situation, we were sorely mistaken. The nurse practitioner confirmed the mass in my left lung; she confirmed the cancer had metastasized and had moved to my liver, stomach, and brain. Also to my lymph nodes. She did not pull any punches. It was Stage IV non-small-cell cancer, a death sentence. She gave the information straightforwardly, but with a calmness that suggested she took no joy in delivering such news. She paused at various intervals to give me a chance to ask questions.

I tried. But my voice was trembling; I had begun to cry, or at least to choke the way I had choked as a little boy when my emotion grew too big for me. Susan ran interference. She asked some clarifying questions, responded to whatever the nurse practitioner said, and handled the farewell at the end of the conversation.

When we were finished, we sat for a while, stunned. There was a great deal we didn't know. Like most cancer patients, we wanted to pin down two things: *How long did I have,* and *How good would the time remaining be?* But those questions, it turned out, were exactly the wrong ones to ask.

For the rest of the day, I received a parade of messages on my phone. My records were being transferred to Dartmouth-Hitchcock, the premier hospital in Lebanon, New Hampshire, a state-of-the-art teaching facility built on the Vermont–New Hampshire border. Susan and I both knew the place; we had both gone there for various small maladies over the years. Friends and relatives, nearly everyone in New Hampshire for that matter, had some association with the hospital. The other option was to go to Boston, or down to New Haven, and we both understood I would not fare well in a city environment. Dartmouth-Hitchcock, architecturally, is a bright, sun-filled facility on a large, rural campus. If I had to be sick, I rationalized, I would remain sick in New Hampshire, the state I loved more than anyplace in the world.

As strange as it is to say it, however, I did not fully accept my diagnosis. Or rather, I refused to accept the *meaning* of the diagnosis. My reluctance was likely a form of mental bargaining, as Dr. Elisabeth Kübler-Ross predicted in her famous statement about the five steps of dying, but I didn't know it yet. The first stage was denial, and while I didn't fully deny the skill of the doctors, or the thoroughness of the tests, I thought, surely, there must be a way around it. Odysseus thinking again, I suppose.

Susan left at the end of the weekend. We said goodbye without any major display of emotions; we had said everything we needed to say, demonstrated our love to each other. It was time to move on and continue with our lives, and we could not spend illimitable hours going over the same thing. Two days remained to prepare for Bob and Ted to arrive. It was also, I realized, the first time I had been alone with the full impact of the diagnosis. On the first night after Susan's absence, I made a fire outside and watched the stars come out. I waited for a large, momentous sweep of feeling to carry me away, but instead I watched the stars appear until I grew tired and thought about going to bed. Besides, having such news, living with it, what did I want to have happen? How could I mark this change? I was keenly aware of artificiality; I did not need to tear at my hair and rend my clothes. No supernatural sign would be unleashed for me to understand that my time on earth was rapidly ending. Death was a quiet thing, I realized. I had never known that. Certainly, death by accident or murder, violent death, would be shocking and painful, but the core of death, the final breath and the retreat into the oblivion that we had lived in before we were born, seemed inevitable and not entirely unwelcome. Watching the wood burn down in my small campfire, I observed how one log burned, became red and fragile, and then, in the end, broke down and returned to the earth. Why I had assumed death was anything different, anything more substantial, puzzled me now. Looking out at the gray water that bordered our property, the tides active, seals sometimes rising on the surface to blow out their air, I knew it was ridiculous to assume my life counted more, meant more, than the death of a gull, or the crunch of a green crab beneath the heel of my water shoe. To accept this transmutation, to go toward death not as a coward, but as a man taking up one last duty, seemed my lot.

# 3

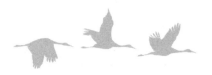

We did not catch any fish to speak of, and after three days of thrashing the water, we determined that it was enough. At the cottage, Bob cut the lawn for me; Ted kept me amused and made dinner. We had drinks on the deck and watched the sea.

Our conversations followed the same pattern I had discovered with my son, Justin. The initial part, the catch-up, as it were, revolved around the latest medical news. I told them my story, explained what I knew. Ted, a retired biology professor, had already done some reading on my diagnosis. His son is a doctor at the Cleveland Clinic in Ohio, so the two together had discussed at length the likely outcome of my situation. It wasn't good, as we all understood, but there was nothing to be done about it.

During my time with my two old friends, I became aware of the subtle danger that a terminal illness carries with it. Namely, I became the center ring of the circus, my body the tent for every conversation. When at last I turned the conversation toward their lives, the answers seemed perfunctory. We all wanted to get back to the main show, this business of dying, and by dissecting it we attempted, I suspect, to disarm it. Or perhaps, more charitably, they both understood that now, in this interval, the everyday concerns of their lives felt diminished, hardly worth talking about in the face of my diagnosis. In many ways, cancer is the trump card that holds sway over all conversations. I would learn in the months to come that telling someone I had cancer — although it was never easy to know when to say it, or how to introduce it — always elicited a solemn expression, a careful word, an acknowledgment that either they had experienced cancer themselves, or someone close to them had died from it. It is, like water, the universal solvent, a topic able to reduce all things to their final elements.

The guys helped me close up the camp, then we took off in three different cars, all of us setting out on the long drive home. It was typical of our departures from fishing camps in the past, except this time I didn't know if I would see them again. After a half century of friendship, we understood we may have said goodbye for the last time. At the very least, it seemed improbable that we would go fishing again the following year.

My first full in-person consultation early the next week was with Dr. Backer, a pulmonary interventionist who had been hired away from Minnesota to head a new Dartmouth department that specialized in illnesses like mine. Susan came with me. She brought a Moleskine journal and sat beside me, ready to take notes. After an LNA read my vital signs and loaded them into my patient portal, Dr. Backer appeared.

He looked young and smart. He looked busy. Covid prevented us from shaking hands, which is an insidious cost that goes largely unrecognized in the tally of the pandemic. Nevertheless, I liked him immediately. So did Susan. He had a calm, gentle nature that first made itself known to us when he asked, haltingly, if anyone had talked to me yet about my situation.

That sounds rather silly in hindsight, but it was a fair question. Yes, people had talked to me, but the truth was, I did not know the boundaries of the land I had just entered. Dr. Backer understood that patients sometimes moved from expert to expert without fully comprehending what had befallen them.

"You're been told you have cancer, yes?" he asked in a soft voice.

"Yes, I have."

"Then you've been told it's grave. I'm going to pull up your CT scan in a moment, but first I want to let you know that it's Stage Four. You were aware of that, I assume."

"Yes."

"In your case, that means it's extremely serious. It is inoperable. Your cancer has spread to your liver and stomach and brain. Your vitals are good otherwise. How is your appetite?"

"Not very strong."

"Let me walk you through it."

Susan took my hand. Dr. Backer pulled up the CT scan I had taken in Plymouth before the fishing trip. He turned the computer screen so that we could both see it. The picture of my chest and lungs looked, frankly, like the images a pregnant couple receives from a sonogram. You knew what you were looking at was important, and human, but it was difficult to ascertain what any of it meant. One thing that jumped out at me was the size of my right lung; it looked swollen and large beside the one on the left. I assumed that was the root of the problem, but it was the opposite.

"If you see here, what you have on your left lung is a pleural effusion. There is always some liquid that serves as a lubricator as your lung inflates and deflates, but in your case you have an overabundance of it in the left cavity."

We both leaned forward. Slowly, the image gained solidity.

"The left lung is compromised. It has folded . . . think of it like a paper bag that may have gotten wet, but then is set out to dry. It doesn't return to its original shape. This is probably the cause of your shortness of breath. You are operating with one good lung. Pressure from the pleural effusion will not allow your left lung to inflate."

The CT scan provided, when all was said and done, a map of my chest — my own sea, so to speak, which had grown wild and turbulent and swollen with rain. He recommended that we remove the liquid as rapidly as possible. I agreed, but then realized he meant now, right away, right here. Cancer, I recognized, seemed to delight in throwing one off balance when it came to timing. Some things progressed rapidly; other developments took much more time.

"I'll wait outside," Susan said after we had asked all the questions we could think up.

Dr. Backer left the room for a few minutes to get some surgical equipment and to enlist the help of a nurse. He told me I could get in a hospital johnny, or simply take off my shirt and wear the johnny in such a way that it could fold forward to allow access to my lungs from behind. This was news to me. In my ignorance, when I thought of lungs I thought of the front side of the body. Not the back. Given a moment to consider it, however, I understood what he proposed. He was going to stick a needle into my left lung and drain it.

"We're going to ask you to sit on the edge of the examining table and lean forward," he instructed when he was ready. "We'll take as much out as we can. Some patients find this uncomfortable. Others are able to tolerate it. You let me know how you're feeling, okay?"

"Okay."

In my mind, this was the true beginning of my illness. The diagnosis, the earlier discussions about symptoms, even the reading Susan and I had done to thread our way through the information, seemed absurdly theoretical in retrospect. This — Dr. Backer swabbing some sort of sanitizing gel on my rib cage halfway down my back — started an assault on my body that would only grow and sharpen in the months to come. Odysseus could not work his way around this. Years before, as a quarterback at Temple University, I had had my knee drained every day before practice. But that memory did not prepare me for the pressure I felt as the needle slipped into my back, dove deeper, probed, and then began to draw out the pleural effusion that sought to impede my lungs. Dr. Backer followed his progress on a sonogram machine. While he worked, he told me that the pleural effusion would return, that we had to schedule a time to insert a catheter, that I would have to learn to drain myself at home, and . . . how did I feel?

"A little light-headed," I said after a while.

"I'd like to get a little more," he said.

"Well, keep going."

I began to sweat, and not long afterward I asked to stop. Dr. Backer encouraged me to take a short break, to not move, and said that I would be more comfortable if he could remove more liquid. We went a little further, then called it a day.

"Sit for a few minutes and recover," he said. "You may cough. Your lung will begin to inflate, and that causes the coughing."

"Will my lung reinflate fully?"

"Hard to say. Probably not all the way."

When I became steady, I thanked Dr. Backer and the nurse then returned to the waiting room to find Susan. I felt like an empty cornhusk. My body understood that something had been removed, and I sensed its absence both as a relief and as a compromise. Something had been taken from me, even if it was merely surplus fluid. I also felt weak and exhausted, something Susan picked up on right away. She held my hand when I told her I needed to sit for a moment. Because we had to walk to the other side of the hospital, she asked if I wanted a wheelchair. I said no, but I wanted to say yes. Mostly, I wanted this all to stop.

• • •

For a couple of days, I felt appreciably lighter. Dr. Backer had removed something like two thousand milliliters from my left lung, which, if I understood it properly, weighed pounds, not simply ounces. I also felt, for the first time, the rounded weight of my retirement. I had been nervous about retirement. I had taught thirty-two years in college, another four or five in high school, and the idea that all my work was behind me, that I had to find a new area of interest, seemed overwhelming in itself. I could continue to write, certainly; I counted on that. I had many books and stories to my credit, but I was now sixty-seven, no longer any kind of player in the world of literature (if I ever had been), and it was difficult to regain the illusion of a younger artist: that what we created was important and *necessary*, that my voice, in the countless chorus of voices that contributed to literature, somehow mattered. Similar to what had occurred in the Mansfield short story, I had depended on the youthful ignorance of self-importance to numb me to the man in the black coat coming to collect his dance. Now in retirement, now with terminal lung cancer, I was supposed to come up with a second act, one that carried with it a concern for human dignity, a righteous sort of occupation that would not wound by its obvious triviality. In preparation, I had undergone CASA (Court Appointed Special Advocates) training throughout the spring, and my plan was to write, work around the house, and do what I could, through CASA, to advocate for overlooked, and often abused, children in New Hampshire. But now, given my physical state, I wondered if I had sufficient time to do much of anything at all.

Summer arrived. It entered softly, warming the land and giving me a few tasks that were nearly beyond my powers. Bring out the porch furniture, put in screens, get the lawn mower running — the work of everyday life. Lifting and moving things into place, I could not catch my breath easily. I became enfeebled, old, slow in my actions. I found bed the most comfortable place to be. My appetite continued to shrink. I knew I was losing weight, but I wasn't sure how much. As I mentioned, I had been on a good eating regimen for the months leading up to my retirement. I had eaten stir-fry, primarily, and stayed far away from sugary carbs. I had lost twenty pounds, but now with cancer grabbing a firmer foothold, weight continued to come off. I had been approximately 220 pounds in late winter; now, just three months later, my weight dropped to 183. I was back to my high school weight.

Dr. Backer scheduled surgery to insert the catheter that would permit me to drain my lung. He said it was not a complicated procedure, which is what one always says when the surgery is happening to someone else. It felt complicated to me, because the image of a semipermanent catheter being inserted into the sheathing around my left lung filled me with dread. The idea of pain did not worry me; it was the fear, I realized, of becoming an invalid, a slice of the man I had been. Many of the things that made summer so appealing involved swimming and water. I was an angler, a swimmer, a kayaker. I knew going into the procedure that I could not get the catheter wet. Infection, especially to my lungs, would bring death faster than I could visualize it, according to the Dartmouth medical staff. The joy of the summer months after the long New England winter had been taken off my calendar.

Dr. Backer was correct. The procedure did not take long. I was given a mild local anesthesia, and in minutes the tip of the catheter entered my lung. It came attached to a long, curled piece of tubing that wound into a spiral and then lay like a coiled serpent on my chest beneath a dura-patch. Susan and Justin came in to the operating room for instructions on how to drain my lung. I was to do it every day; the pleural effusion, we had come to learn, was a killer. The faster it could be drawn off, the better. I was to keep track of the amount drained each day. Unless the effusion subsided, which would mean I had improved or the cancer was in remission, the catheter was now a permanent part of my life.

Coming home that day from the hospital, I had difficulty standing erect. The incision hurt. My body no longer felt inviolate; I had surrendered autonomy over what could be done to me. I didn't doubt that Dr. Backer and the others had my best interests in mind, but I also wondered what price I was willing to pay. My mother had died of cancer when I was eighteen; my father had died in his seventies from a heart attack, the direct result of chemotherapy. During the fall of my first year in college, I had seen my mother wither and become empty of all life. I had carried her down the stairs on her last Christmas. I was young and steady on my feet, happy to provide a service, but nothing had prepared me for her lack of weight. I carried her illness.

Now it was my time. I went to bed in the early afternoon and felt as if the cancer had already won. Justin configured a handle that he dangled from a beam above my bed so that I might lift and shift my weight. It also provided me with a boost up when I needed to go to the bathroom. Although I was grateful for the improvements to my environment, I was acutely conscious that we were building a sickroom around me. That night I ate a few spoonsful of yogurt and fell asleep at sundown.

Nonetheless, I did not feel despairing. Not entirely. Gradually, I had abandoned the idea of Odysseus's cleverness and tried to fill its place with a muted stoicism. I had long turned to *Meditations* by Marcus Aurelius during trying periods in my life, but I had done so with the assurance that I did not have to wrestle with my mortality. Marcus Aurelius, an old man himself when he sat down and composed his guide to life, had implored me — and his many readers — to consider and weigh our own endings, but it had always felt like an academic exercise, a thought experiment that titillated by its imagining of death while not taking our own short life span to heart. Now I realized that *Meditations* exactly mirrored my thinking. This life, my imminent death, had suddenly become the sharpest flame in the torch, and Marcus Aurelius knew the path I was soon to take.

I was also aware, acutely aware, of how fortunate I had been in life and how rich my days were even after the diagnosis. I had a son. I had a home, paid off, and enough medical coverage to shield me from excessive costs. I had sufficient money in the bank and friends and family who cared about me. I did not have a list of unmet challenges or delights. I had traveled, enjoyed myself, hiked and kayaked where I liked, fished streams in Wyoming's Wind River Range, fished New Zealand, lived in Vienna, hiked inn-to-inn in the Windermere Lake District, biked France, Holland, and England, biked Nova Scotia's Cabot Trail, served in the Peace Corps in West Africa, run a dogsled team, written novels and short stories, rafted the Grand Canyon, visited the Great Barrier Reef, pretended to hold up a horizontal redwood tree for a silly photo in California then stayed to absorb the sense of the forest, experienced a lovely boyhood filled with games and laughter; I did not have anything left unsaid. I had enjoyed good relations with my students, given them a fair effort, I hoped, and retired with a solid body of work behind me. If as a young boy I could have forecast how I wanted my life to go, it would largely have followed the path I had actually lived. I was lucky in my health and lucky in my daily life. I had no complaints.

And most important, I had Susan. It was Susan whose hand I held at night; it was Susan who lay her head on my chest to listen to my lungs, thinking that she could judge them by sheer love and attentiveness. It was Susan who kissed me, refused to kid me along, helped me look squarely at things without catastrophizing them. She did research; she brought me food and tried to get me to eat. She went out and purchased a new digital thermometer so that she could scout for fever. She also listened to me when I told her that I wasn't sure I wanted to see this all to the very end. Suicide, death with dignity, was very much on my mind, and Susan listened without alarm, admitting that were the situation reversed, she might make the same determination.

That's where things stood when we met Dr. Dragnev, the oncologist assigned to my case. An MD from the Higher Institute of Medicine in Sofia, Bulgaria, he had worked at Baylor College of Medicine in Houston, Texas; the National Cancer Institute in Bethesda, Maryland; and the Memorial Sloan Kettering Cancer Center in New York City. He had been at Dartmouth from 1999, and although we didn't know it at the time, he was known to cancer patients and their families throughout Vermont and New Hampshire. He was known not only for his medical knowledge but, more importantly, for his kindness. If you could call up a doctor from central casting, Dr. Dragnev fit the bill. It was hard to guess his age, but his hair was gray and kept short. He had the tired demeanor of a man who has seen a great deal, has been asked to do much, and now approached life evenly. He spoke softly, but always with a light of humor in his eyes. His job was serious, deadly serious, but he brought to it a human understanding that we are in this together, that the healthy are a step away from trading places with the sick, that medicine is at least partially a coaching practice. Susan and I liked him immediately. It was a pleasure, actually, to be in his company.

On our first visit, we reviewed the entire situation. I had the sense that a universe of information rested behind his comments. As adults, we believe we understand how the world is constructed, what governs it, but in the first minutes of our conversation I realized Dr. Dragnev knew my circumstances, and the likely outcomes of each potential treatment, better than I ever would. Working without referring to a computer screen — he had seen my condition a thousand times before, I imagined — he explained various options open to me. Susan took particularly sharp notes, but I felt slightly at sea. Chemotherapy seemed to be the recommended course of action. Without it, without something entering the picture to curtail the growth of the cancer, I was on an extremely short plank. Chemotherapy, however, scared me more than cancer; I had seen its effects on friends and family who had endured it, and the slow whittling away of my body, the acceptance of profound nausea in order to live an undetermined amount of time in a cloudy future, struck me as a bad bargain.

"What if I did nothing?" I asked after we had talked awhile.

"You would not last long," he answered, raising his eyebrows.

"How long?"

He smiled. This was and is the central question on all cancer patients' minds. He had doubtlessly heard it many times before, and he was prepared to answer it.

"If any oncologist gives you an answer to that question, you have a bad oncologist."

"But you can surely give me some idea. A rough estimate, anyway . . ."

"I could give you statistics and averages, but they are meaningless to individual cases. Yes, it will be sooner than it would be without the cancer, but the fact is you have the cancer. Who can say? It's not a good idea to focus on the time left to you. Focus on how you feel and how you want to live."

I wasn't sure I bought this. I certainly put it on a mental list to revisit. After all, if you are going on a trip, wouldn't you want to know if it would take ten minutes or ten years? Didn't I need to know what to plan, what to pack (to follow the trip metaphor), what kind of trials I might encounter? It seemed somewhat unfeeling on his part to be dismissive of my request for this kind of knowledge. Later I learned that Dr. Dragnev did not issue time declarations because, among other things, he worried that they would become self-fulfilling. Tell a patient they have a year to live, and that's where they set their goalpost. True, also, for a shorter time. It was more useful — and I would come to agree with him, although it took time to see it — to concentrate on the present, on how I felt today.

Near the end of our consultation, he offered to set up an appointment with the Dartmouth palliative care team. I wasn't even sure of the definition of *palliative*, although I surmised it was something to do with comfort at the end of life. I said yes, I would love to talk to that team, although I was shocked to find myself that close to a last call. Only truly sick people spoke to the palliative team, I supposed, which was, if I understood properly, the conduit to hospice and eventual death.

That was it. We shook hands, although he made us use a gel cleaner immediately afterward. He went off to see his next patient. Susan and I walked back through the hospital, dazed, rocky, unsure of everything except our trust in Dr. Dragnev. We both commented that he was a good man, one who made us feel human and heard. As we left, we passed through the waiting room of the cancer ward, although it was not known by that name. Whereas before I might have spotted people who were sick, or had apparent deficits, now I saw them as brave humans asked to endure more than they should. I was part of their number now, and although I could still walk well, still think and eat and laugh, we were the toys in the chest that were broken. And we all knew it.

# 4

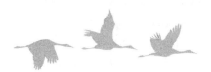

I had been a lifelong reader, but during the summer days around visits with Dr. Backer and Dr. Dragnev, I read as I had not read in years. Some of it, likely, was the fact that I had more time on my hands. As a teacher, I had spent years reading student work. One of the promises I made to myself was that in retirement I would read exactly what I wanted to read. Further, the commotion of daily life, the busyness of doing, dropped off sharply due to my illness. My body had betrayed me, but my mind — at least as far as we knew — felt healthy and sharp and hungry.

It did not seem to matter what I read. I read Robert Parker mysteries, Dick Francis mysteries, western tales from Larry McMurtry, a story about the Yankees versus Red Sox rivalry, a National Book Award finalist called *The Big House*, *Frankenstein*, a memoir of a Blasket Island (Irish) nurse, articles in *The New Yorker*, short stories online, Marcus Aurelius, an epistolary novel about bog people, an experimental novel by Doris Lessing revolving around her parents. And more. I had a very short fuse with books; I could not tolerate fluff or literary pretense. I was keenly interested in stories, in genuine voice, but if a book struck me as false, or preening for sophistication, I traded it at the local Goodwill store for something more to my taste.

I also gained an appetite for YouTube tutorials. I wanted to know more about medieval masonry, about the Constitution, about the workings of the Supreme Court, about barrel making, rockweed, house design, shark attacks, courtroom behavior. Much of it was silly and hardly germane to my situation, but a good deal of it filled in lacunae in my knowledge. I spent a happy day watching Napoleon documentaries, never before understanding the connection between the first Napoleon and the second, the French aggression of the early nineteenth century and the later misadventures against Prussia. I was not hurried in these short lessons. All knowledge, all books, seemed worth investigating, and I paged through them like a prospective wedding couple sampling slices of wedding cake from a caterer's display table.

I also read some of my own work, a curiosity I had been reluctant to satisfy through most of my adult life. I had first published a novel in 1981; it was now 2021, forty years later. Yes, I had occasionally gone back to look at my own work — usually when it somehow fell into my lap, a spontaneous short read to confirm something I had said or thought — but now I had time to assess the value of my effort. Call it a literary selfie. What had I been doing all these years? Did the books stand up to time? Was the artistry I hoped to bring to their composition still evident, if it had ever been evident, after a decade or more? The avidity and ambition I had felt years ago, the desire to write, to produce novels and stories, had it been worthwhile?

Let's say this: I found I did not hate what I had done, and for that I felt grateful. Some of the works seemed to come out just right, or at least as close to my initial vision for them as was desirable. Other works seemed trivial. From the vantage of someone with terminal cancer, I would not write them again. But I had been making a living, too, and I had written for a roof above me and food on the table, so I forgave myself some of my missteps and shortcomings. The good and the bad. It was all part of a life. I felt at peace with the work I attempted, and that seemed a solid, good thing.

Meanwhile, Susan, Justin, and I sat down at our dining room table to have a Zoom conference with the palliative team a few days after meeting with Dr. Dragnev. I did not think a great deal about it beforehand. I was not *that* sick, I told myself. I was not there yet. The meeting was, I felt, a chance to get to know the team well before I would need it. In my health bank account, these were funds I would not need for some time.

We met with Dr. Rachel E. Gaidys, a palliative care physician with a Vermont background. She explained that I was officially a patient of Dr. Maxwell Vergo and that he would come on later in the conversation to fill in anything we had failed to touch upon. For now, she said, she simply wanted to talk, to get a sense of where I was in my thinking.

"What's important to you as you go forward?" she asked in a warm, kind voice. "Can you tell me a little about who you are?"

I'm not sure why, but the question paralyzed me. Speaking around a plug of deep emotion, my throat unable to form words readily, I said something about wanting to be outside, to be part of nature . . .

And then I began to cry.

To Dr. Gaidys's everlasting credit, she did not offer any phony words of cheer or consolation. I was dying; that was the unavoidable truth. She sat quietly, listening for the words I could utter when I was able again to speak. Susan held my hand. My son held my hand. Dr. Gaidys listened as Dr. Dragnev and Dr. Backer had listened. They wanted me to have dignity; they wanted the choices I made to reflect whomever I was before the cancer had entered my life.

Gradually, I was able to talk, but my thoughts were poorly formed. Who thinks concretely about how they want to be treated as they prepare to die? I certainly hadn't. I was interested in life, not death, and so her patient demeanor did more to unsettle me than nearly any conversation I had up until that point. She was inscrutable. It became obvious that this was not her first time in a conversation of this nature.

When it was her time to speak, she reassured me regarding some central concerns. She said it sounded as if I would prefer to die at home, not in a hospital bed, and that she could guarantee that they could make me comfortable. Dying, in other words, would not hurt. She promised that the hospice team affiliated with Dartmouth was excellent and that I had nothing to fear once I was in its capable hands. Hearing that, I felt better. I had not thought a great deal about pain, but I imagined it could be terrible if things went the wrong way. It was a relief to put that concern behind me.

"When should we contact hospice?" Susan asked, her pen poised over her black notebook. It was a note-taking question, merely a request for information.

"Tomorrow," Dr. Gaidys said without a moment's hesitation, her voice calm, the shock of that timeline, that speed, taking our tongues from our mouths.

Somewhere along here we began playing Fan Tan. It was a card game my family had grown up on. Its appeal is its simplicity. The object is to get rid of all your cards by playing them in sequence, and by suit, before your opponents get rid of theirs. The game begins by someone playing a seven, then the next person plays the eight, the six, or another seven, and so on until you arrive at the king on one end and the ace at the other. If you have a play, you must play. You pass if you don't have a play, and thereby start to lag behind. The game requires some strategy, not a great deal, and gives the players ample time to kibitz. As we scored it in my family, three points are awarded to the winner, two to the second-place finisher, and one for the loser.

We played on the porch of my home, Justin, Susan, and I, usually in the late afternoons when the day had begun to cool and the sunlight swept away to the west. The game was demanding enough to be interesting, but simple enough to allow our losses to be blamed on bad cards. You could force the other players into filling out your desired suit, but only up to a point, and only if the game tilted in your favor.

We were on the porch playing one early evening when Dr. Dragnev called and asked to speak to me. I turned my cards upside down on the table and took the call. We exchanged a few pleasantries, then he informed me that, thanks to a blood test he had ordered, I had matched a treatment based on a drug called Tagrisso, a product of AstraZeneca Labs. It turned out that I had a relatively rare EFGR gene mutation, more common in Asian men, but one that meant, on the upside, I would live longer than anticipated. It also meant that I would no longer need chemotherapy; I would take a single pill each morning with food, and although the cancer would not be vanquished, I stood a good chance of impeding or retarding the cancer growth so that I could resume at least a part of my life.

"So no more discussions of not taking a treatment," Dr. Dragnev said, his voice on the phone sounding firm. "This is what you will do, all right?"

"Yes, yes, thank you," I replied, my eyes going immediately to Susan's to let her see that the news was good.

"Okay, I will order it on this end. It's expensive, and I'm not sure how much Medicare covers, but you have no choice."

"Thank you, Doctor. Thank you so much."

As soon as I hung up, I hugged Susan and Justin. It was miraculous news, and it sent us all to our phones to look up Tagrisso, gene mutations, mean life span on the pill, and so on. I knew it was good news, but I didn't truly have a notion, at that point, how outstanding it was. No chemotherapy. A good chance of remission. Yes, I was still a sick man, still draining my lung on a regular basis, but my horizon had just brightened tenfold from where I had been prior to the call. I did not have to die by summer's end. Through Dr. Dragnev's good management, and through the wonder of a single pill, I was given time, a good pocketful of time, and I had escaped the anguish of chemotherapy, at least for the moment. It seemed incomprehensible.

It was only later, and gradually, that I understood what the pill meant and how it had changed my perspective. I was reminded of the story and play *Flowers for Algernon*, in which a man with mental limitations is given a treatment that, temporarily, increases his aptitude in every direction. I read the story long ago with a high school class. The discussion point, I remembered, had been whether ethically it was fair to administer such a regimen to the man if the researchers knew, in advance, that the treatment would gradually lose its efficacy, and the patient would return to his former level of intelligence. Would he then have the pain of remembering what he once was but was no longer? How could the patient reconcile his final state with the increased intelligence he had experienced? Would it be better, we wondered as a group, to leave well enough alone and allow the patient to accommodate himself to his circumstances and make his peace with that?

That was the flip side of the Tagrisso miracle. Yes, I would improve, but it was impossible to say for how long or to what level. At any point the medicine could begin to fail, and then I would be back in my former position, this time without a great deal of hope, the tides or winds or whatever we wanted to call it reversing and reclaiming the land it had lost. Hope, I realized, could be a heartless thing, and one fed it, if one were wise, with grave caution.

# 5

The question of time continued to haunt me. With Susan's help, I consulted graphs and statistics that documented the Tagrisso bump, as we called it. It quickly became clear that the increased longevity many patients experienced was not an illusion; it was not imaginary or inflated for sales. Tagrisso worked. Now in its third generation, Tagrisso was a cancer patient's best hope in many instances. In fact, Susan's mother, Nancy, attended — virtually — the funeral of her college roommate who had succumbed finally, in her eighties, to cancer. When a mutual friend gave a short talk about the woman's life, she mentioned that act three of their departed friend's journey had been the ten years she lived on Tagrisso. Coming out of nowhere as it did, that news filled us with hope. Maybe I had ten years! If I lived ten years in reasonable fashion, that meant I could be seventy-seven when I died. That seemed a fair bargain. Tagrisso was the proverbial cat's paw, the severed feline limb used to rake chestnuts out of a burning brazier.

Psychologically, however, I could not trust the good turn my treatment had taken. My son ordered the Tagrisso from the Dartmouth specialty pharmacy, but I was still as sick as I had been before the good news. Every second evening at five thirty, my son drained my lung. That schedule had been approved by Dr. Backer. Putting on a mask, a pair of gloves, my son knelt before me and slowly peeled back the bandage that held the catheter. My great fear was that he would somehow forget the nest of catheter tubing that connected to my lung, and in the stickiness of the bandage he would tug and rip or twist the needle in my chest. As a result, I was sometimes short with him, telling him to go carefully, while he evinced nothing but the kindest patience and care as my nurse. Susan, too, worked beside him, and together they watched and coordinated their movements as Justin connected the tube to the vacuum bottle that sucked the yellowish liquid from my chest. We coded the effusion's color by types of beer. We had amber pilsner draws and darker, brown ale draws. We could never anticipate what would flow out of my lung. During the first week or two of the procedure, we did not understand the complete workings of the bottles, so that, hooking me up, we sometimes drained too rapidly, taking my breath as the lung reinflated without the liquid to hold it captive. The feeling in my chest in these moments reminded me of summer days as a boy when I had been too long in a chlorinated pool. My lungs burned slightly, and the breath I took seemed borrowed and not completely mine.

How long was a man likely to live if he drained his chest every other day? I could not reconcile the idea of Tagrisso coming in as a cavalry charge to save my life with the decrepit older man who looked in the mirror and saw a skeletal figure gazing back, a translucent coil of tubing taped to his chest, his body clearly asking for something it could not find. My appetite continued to betray me. I ate yogurt and bananas. I drank lemonade, grateful for the sharp piquancy of the lemons. I had always had a devilish sweet tooth, but even my favorite treats could not tempt me beyond a few bites. My throat was often scratchy and dry, making it difficult to swallow. I felt I was living in the type of movie that shows the ending first, then slowly fills in the why and how of the story. I had seen my ending; it was now only a matter of time until the plot points carried me to the inevitable conclusion.

In addition to my mistrust of Tagrisso's promise, I felt my internal compass turning softly to find a new bearing. It became apparent to me that most of us live with a stream of activity that, as much as we may complain about it, insulates and silences the mortal voice that is there to speak to us if we take the time to hear it. Before my diagnosis, I had been searching, like most people, for the next thing, the next activity, the item I might purchase, the trip I would take, the people I would meet, the foods I could try. In the space of a little more than a month, the constancy of that forward thrust had suddenly calmed. Imagine a boat that had been traveling at a good speed. When the engine is cut, the world becomes silent and the wake falls forward and captures the boat. Susan, who has long been a fan of the Austrian philosopher Rudolf Steiner and quotes him often, has always said that children live in a dream until they slowly wake from it, sometimes by harsh reality, sometimes by the early introduction of media or video games that insult the child with their over-stimulation. Likewise, she quotes Steiner as saying the elderly return to the dream of their childhood, letting things go, slowly reentering a world that is internal and personal and very much like a world inside a world. Although I do not think I fully entered Steiner's dream, I did glimpse it; I felt its reassurance, the idea that those things that seemed to matter no longer influenced my life. To hear people speak about vacations coming up, or what they planned to do with the summer, made me nod and smile, but I did not go with them in their thinking. I wished them well. I had no sense of leaving them, but only of going to a world that I understood and no longer needed to explain to anyone.

Loss is the price we pay for life, I have read. It is our fate to lose everything if we live long enough. In a blink I had lost the ability to hike, to ride a bike, to swim, to plan. Yes, our society applauds people who fight cancer — or any grave illness — and frequently employs the language of sports or war to speak about defeating the wolf at the door. I received many notes and emails that told me that the sender knew I would fight and beat this dread disease. And although I understood they meant well by the exhortations, I also knew they were fooling themselves. Naturally, we could do our best, resist when sensible, follow the dictates of our doctors, but this was not a contest in which I wanted to engage. I did not hate the prospect of death or see it as an enemy. The dream metaphor was a more coherent approach for me. The dream would come eventually, but the moment of its arrival, the strength of its welcome fog, was still to be determined.

I began taking Tagrisso in midsummer, the warnings surrounding the pill sharp and loud. The side effects could be intolerable: diarrhea, acne, numbness, "Tagrisso hair," stomach upset, and so forth. Each individual reacts differently, of course, but I was made to understand that the drug contained potent chemicals. The preferred method of consumption was to spill a pill out into the bottle cap, pop it in my mouth, and swallow it as quickly as possible. I was to guard against touching it with my hand. If I did so, I was encouraged to wash my fingers to rid them of contaminants. I was also instructed to swallow the pill back in my mouth, thereby protecting my lips and tongue to whatever degree was possible. In short, I was to be on alert; the pill, while certainly an ally against my cancer, could also turn traitorous.

The effects of the Tagrisso could also affect my bones, so I was scheduled to receive a monthly shot of bone density medicine (Prolia; Xgeva) in the fatty triceps area of my arm. For my first dose, I entered the infusion center at Dartmouth, where cancer patients sat in large recliners and endured the medical drip attached to their arms or chest catheters. It was a quiet place. Like a library, people spoke in soft voices, perhaps honoring the rest needed by the patients who sometimes dozed while their blood was fruitfully poisoned. I had visited infusion centers before with loved ones, but I had never considered myself a candidate for one of those yielding recliners. Now, however, I was told by a nurse to sit and relax. The medicine prescribed for me had to be warmed. I sat in a comfortable chair, pulled a magazine onto my lap, and waited.

Almost immediately a bird feeder set up outside the window distracted me in the loveliest way possible. It's easy to make too much of these interludes, to lend them too much meaning, but for me, in that instant, I felt I had a known companion, many of them, to help. I had always loved birds and always had a feeder throughout the New Hampshire winters, and seeing them here, chickadees, house sparrows, titmice, and cardinals, brought moisture to my eyes. The world is made of small moments, and here, providentially, the birds had come to visit with me. I watched them with keen interest. Had I ever seen exactly the black cap of the chickadee before? Had I noticed previously the birds' talons or claws, the grasping way they clung to the feeder bars? And what about the corvid triangle on the cardinal's head? How did anything in nature grow so red?

It was an easy moment to dismiss as pure romanticization of what nature meant to me, but it was nevertheless true that I hung on the sight of the birds flitting back and forth. They lifted me. Perhaps, I realized, that one of the few gifts that cancer brought was the lens of looking closer. Without time, time's importance grew and demanded attention. I thought of Emily's speech in Thornton Wilder's *Our Town*, that most

New-Hampshire-ish of New Hampshire works, when she at last accepts death and begins back to her grave. Turning once more to Grover's Corners and her parents, she says goodbye to clocks ticking, to new ironed dresses, to food, to hot baths and her butternut tree, to sleep, to waking from sleep, to coffee. She asks the stage manager if anyone living ever truly realizes the beauty of life while they live it, and the stage manager answers immediately, *Saints and poets, maybe, they do some.*

I was neither a saint nor a poet, but I was a writer, and my art had depended on my ability to observe. Sitting in the chair, the slow beat of dripping machines nearby, the occasional squeak of a nurse's shoes scuffing the linoleum, the whir of birds' wings stirring the air beside the pine that supported the feeder, I felt, at least, that that specific ability could not be taken from me. The eyes are the last to die; they do not need to produce energy to function but merely take in what the light of the world sends to them. I promised myself that I would see to the last and that I would make whatever effort I could to collect as much beauty as my eyes could find.

To hold my pills, I rehabbed an old wooden box that had been hanging around the house forever. It was a shabby-looking thing, but I refused to entertain a standard "pill box" with the days of the week gaily stamped on each cube of medicine. For me, a pill box signified old age and weariness, a fussiness that descended on us as we grew older. A beat-up wooden box seemed more suited to someone who could still go fishing if he had a mind to do it.

I took three pills every morning, one of which was the magic genie, Tagrisso. The other two were simple vitamins, calcium mostly, to feed my weakened bones. My son set an alarm on my phone that went off every day at nine forty-five. At ten I gulped down the pills on a tide of orange juice or apple cider. I made sure my belly was full beforehand, usually by consuming a banana and a muffin. Frankly, eating no longer concerned me; I could eat anything and not gain weight, which was a sly side benefit, I suppose, of combating cancer. A dubious superpower. The only one I've ever brushed up against.

While waiting to see what the Tagrisso would do, how much, if any, of my life I could reclaim, I gave myself the autumn off. I told people I had earned it. I had spent close to forty years in the classroom, so I was due for a good break. In my gut, however, I knew a second truth: that I had grown hesitant and tentative. I was not doing much, a fact of which I was well aware, but I also did not have much interest in the world around me. I still followed the news and listened to reports of daily activity from family members or from Susan, but I stood back and gave myself permission and distance to be sick. Honestly, I was not incapacitated regarding daily life. The dreaded side effects of Tagrisso did not land on me. My bowels remained stable; I did not sprout acne or feel nauseated at mealtimes. As a matter of fact, after a fortnight on Tagrisso, I began to feel better. Much better. My appetite returned stage by stage, meal by meal, until, at one family dinner, I ordered a personal pizza and a dark ale. Furthermore, the lung effusion that had so readily filled up the vacuum bottles my son had connected to my tube gradually began to diminish. I asked Dr. Dragnev if that meant I could get the catheter removed, and he told me to wait awhile. The final decision, he added, was Dr. Backer's to make.

Part of my difficulty in regaining a level of activity in my life, I realized, revolved around the fact that I had not stepped solidly into my retirement. Whatever transition one typically made upon retirement had been eclipsed, by many levels of magnitude, by the cancer. Furthermore, the perennial time problem centered itself in my brain and filled me with caution. How did you plan to do X if you did not know, for instance, whether you would require hospitalization? Could you travel in my condition, regardless of the Covid pandemic that seemed to surge in early fall? Was it fair to take on a CASA case, for example, if I could not predict how well I would be by the time the case came to court?

It turned out — although it sounds like a stupid bumper sticker — that I was living to die, not dying to live. Sloppy and simplistic, but true. When my friend Bob called and asked me if I was interested in going up to the Deboullie Mountain area of Maine to a fishing camp called Red River, I did not give a definitive answer right away. I knew the place because we had visited it before, so that was not an obstacle. Moreover, I loved the aesthetic of Red River. It was a throwback camp set in the North Woods recreational area of Maine, where the townships frequently are not named but merely numbered. It was beyond cell reception, beyond electricity. The accommodations consisted of small cabins with gas lights and wood or gas stoves set beside Island Pond, a small water body packed with trout. Meals were served family-style in the main lodge, and the food, I knew, was excellent. Bob told me that he had reserved a special cabin on an island in the center of the pond, a place that would require us to paddle in to dinner and breakfast, four trips, minimum, each day. Two other guys, Jim and Tim, were going along. It's possible that we had the most boring names imaginable — Joe, Bob, Tim, and Jim — of any group ever assembled for an outing.

At my next monthly visit to Dartmouth-Hitchcock, I asked Dr. Dragnev if it was all right to go fishing.

"Do you like to go fishing?" he asked with his wonderful accent.

As usual, his question was more loaded than I at first understood.

"Yes, but it's pretty remote."

"If you were going somewhere truly remote, then I would say no. But if you can drive to a hospital or get medical attention in a few hours, then I would say you're fine to go."

"Probably three or four hours to a hospital."

He shrugged. His clear message: *It's your decision to make.*

I found this little standoff interesting. I wondered what I wanted him to say. *No, don't go, don't ever leave your home.* Of course I needed to be careful, needed to be smart, but I couldn't spend whatever time I had left trying to insulate myself for . . . what? What was the thing, the event, the moment I had to experience that made it prudent to forgo whatever pleasure I could have in order to live another safe day? At what point was it life-reducing to be so cautious? It wasn't easy to know. I had once departed for three years to West Africa with little more than a duffel bag, and I had hitchhiked around the country several times with a backpack and a hundred bucks in my wallet, but now, at sixty-seven, I was asking for permission to go fishing. Cancer, I slowly realized, was a mental assault as much as it was a physical one.

On a beautiful Friday in September, I drove to northern Maine, entering Deboullie Township — Deboullie is an Americanization of the French geological term *d'eboulis*, or talus slope — and the northern Maine recreational area known on maps as T15 R9. I traveled logging roads and followed small, hand-painted signs for Red River Camps. It took awhile. Finally, however, I pulled into the camp area, the pond bright and welcoming. This was, I remembered, the kind of place I had always loved. The pond itself was beautiful, and the cabins, constructed of brown logs, did their best to remain hidden. Jen, the owner, and Gloria, the camp cook, welcomed me with hugs. Bob, Tim, and Jim pulled in behind me. We had three days to fish in spectacular water, all of it in some of the most primitive land east of the Mississippi.

We unloaded the contents of our cars into two canoes. Bob and I took one, Jim and Tim the other. It was late afternoon by the time we landed on the island at the center of the pond. From what Jen and Gloria had related, the island cabin was the oldest at Red River Camps. It was a stout little building, propped amid the gnarled roots of weathered pines, brown and musty, a perfect setting for a fishing trip. The interior of the camp held a picnic table, a gas stove, and a sleeping loft. Although we were all roughly the same age, the boys insisted that I take the prime bedroom, one that did not require me to climb a ladder or hoist myself up on a top bunk. While I had always had a conception of myself as a rough-and-ready fellow, the last individual to require special accommodations, now, in the space of a month or two, I was given the privilege afforded to the sick and infirm. It had an effect similar to being called sir for the first few times. If these men saw me as weakened, a wobbly cancer patient, who was I to disagree?

After settling in, we decided to fish our way slowly back to the main lodge where we could expect a warm dinner waiting for us. The last time we had visited, in a spring a few seasons back, Bob and I had seen trout rising all day. Now, at this stage in the fall, we spotted few rises. Jen had warned that the fishing was not great; she had said people were having little luck. We listened with half an ear. We had confidence in our abilities, and besides, we knew the pond held thousands of fish. Dumb luck, we reasoned, would provide if our skill would not.

We caught a few, none of them large. Nonetheless, it was wonderful to be out. The leaves had started to turn and some of the buildings — an old boathouse, especially — lent the camp a classic New England feeling. We existed in a calendar page. We gathered no noise except the sound of our own voices or the whip of a fly line stretching for a cast. I was reminded that few activities gave me as much sustainable joy as fly fishing. The bonus of fishing with my friend Bob, whom I had known for more than a half century, reassured me that I had made the correct decision about coming. If I was going to ask my eyes to capture beauty, then I needed to make trips like these and not rule them out in deference to cancer.

Except that I had a cough.

At first it felt as if I had gotten on the wrong side of pollen or dust or even woodsmoke. It was an annoying cough, shallow and unproductive, but fairly constant. Think of an elderly aunt or uncle in the next bedroom coughing politely, but relentlessly, their attempts to stifle the noise of their hacking making you lift your head from the pillow to question if they needed help. Usually, we think we can control our bodily functions, at least to some degree, but the cough would not rest. The thought passed through my mind that this was cancer announcing itself once again. The good feelings I had experienced less than an hour before suddenly seemed to mock me. Now instead of commending myself for being willing to adventure out on a small excursion, I was suddenly asking myself what in the world I was doing — with Stage IV lung cancer — on a pond in remote, unbelievably remote, Maine.

The cough persisted through an excellent dinner and grew stronger on the paddle back to our cabin. Bob asked several times if I was all right and I told him I was. But I did not feel all right. The cough pecked at me; I felt, too, that I was surely a distraction on such a quiet water body. My angling companions had to weigh my cough against the diagnosis they had heard about. I saw the doubt in their eyes. *How was this going to end?* they seemed to wonder.

I had difficulty sleeping that night and twice woke to find myself dangerously short of breath. The cough continued. I took an over-the-counter bronchial dilator, hoping that would reduce the phlegm that threatened to choke me, but it made no difference. For the first time since I had been diagnosed, I was frightened. I couldn't discern if this was the beginning of something extremely worrisome — a cancer attack, if such a thing were possible — or part of an ongoing illness that I would have to endure from this point forward. A great deal about cancer — about experiencing cancer, that is to say — was like a boggy water crossing. You thought you knew what was underfoot, but you could be disastrously mistaken.

The next morning the cough was no better. In fact, my chest had tightened during the night. I studied the boys to see how my coughing had affected them. They did their best to ignore my hacking, and they showed me every kindness, but we all had to pretend that it wasn't a thing. Cancer guy in Maine with a never-ending cough; it didn't bode well.

I faced my second night in the cabin with genuine fear. Several times the night before I had dozed off and then had woken to a clogged congestion in my lungs so murky that I had difficulty breathing. I wondered if it was possible simply to lose the ability to draw in air. Pipes and exhaust systems became bound up, certainly, so why not a human respiratory system? Most of us live our days assuming we can shake things off, continue going regardless of the internal trouble — we would fold many times throughout a life if we didn't have that inherent resilience — but it was possible, I now realized, that I could die from respiratory failure. One of the breaths I tried to take might not come, I sensed, and if it faltered, I wondered if I would pass out somehow, or simply die choking.

Gloomy thoughts. I felt terrible telling Bob that I needed to leave the next morning after a second breathless night. Because he is a fine man, and a friend of fifty years, he stated that he would go with me. The beauty of his response was that he did not hesitate. If his friend was sick, to hell with the fishing trip. It was Bob's way and always had been.

We left after breakfast and drove south and east to Houlton, Maine, where the emergency room in the local hospital was empty. A nurse took me in, recorded my vitals, asked me fifty questions about my cancer diagnosis. They recommended X-rays and a CT scan, but I told them I had just had a CT scan less than a week before. After conferring away from me, they sent in a respiratory therapist with a nebulizer, a funny, foggy flute that gave me a warm, healing breath. I immediately felt better. The cough paused for the first time in days. The doctor on call came in, went over my symptoms, talked to me for a while about my cancer protocols, then prescribed a regimen of antibiotics. It seemed I had an infection in my lungs, one of the keenest threats to my hopes of living a few years with cancer, and he suggested I not delay in returning to my regular oncology team.

Afterward Bob and I ate a hamburger in a nearby café, booked a room in an adjoining motel, and called it a day. I needed to rest. A little later we lay on our two beds and watched the Red Sox, who were having an unexpectedly strong season. While I talked to Bob and made observations about different players, a second part of my mind remained occupied with what had just occurred. True, the nebulizer and the antibiotics had already begun to work, but what did it say about my readiness to travel or even to live? I was of two minds: On one side, I had managed the crisis and I was none the worse for wear. Yes, I had cut into my friend's vacation, but that couldn't really be helped. On the other hand, I could not rid myself of the memory of the inability to breathe. That memory did not diminish or wash away despite feeling better now that I had undergone medical treatment. I had been unable to breathe, had been unable to force air through the deep cobweb of infection and pulmonary effusion. Sitting up in bed back in the cabin, alone in the early-morning darkness, I had opened my mouth like a fish gasping for air, and the air did not reach me, the air could not penetrate the pearled cocoon of my cancerous body.

# 6

It is easy to become self-absorbed when you receive a diagnosis like the one I had received, but it is also, to a large degree, unfair to the people closest to us. I'll give a small example. While I was on the fishing trip with my friends, my son, Justin, came into our house after sunset and, because he had been out all day, no lights were on to help him. Especially after the diagnosis, I would typically be home, a few lights on, maybe a fire going in the fireplace, or maybe some sort of dinner cooking, but on this particular night the house was dark and quiet. Later Justin told me that he experienced a painful moment: He had stepped inside and realized, almost for the first time, that this empty house was waiting, that I would be gone sooner than later, that he would be a son without a father. It hit him. He told me he stood for a moment, teary, and did not turn on a light immediately. We had been so caught up — he had been so caught up — in the management of my illness that he had not absorbed the central fact of the situation: I was dying and he would be alone in the not-too-distant future. He had to adapt to the new reality, mostly on his own, without the attendant fuss of people asking if he was all right.

Susan, likewise, contended with the knowledge that this person in her life, a friend, a lover, and a companion, was not going to be the man to accompany her into her own old age. I was getting off the train, and she would have to finish the remainder of the journey on her own. That was not a small understanding to gain, and yet she could not speak of it, really, without nudging her loss ahead of my death. It's not that we were afraid or too timid to talk about it. It was merely that no real good might come of it. It was a bald fact, a reality that many women involved with older men experience. Unfairly, she would see me to my ending, making it more comfortable and kinder than it could possibly be without her, but then she would be on her own again, while I ducked out for a doughnut.

Somewhere in early fall she began wearing my gray, cable-knit sweater, manufactured by J. Crew. It was a good sweater, warm as a goat, and she told me it was not scratchy, a thing she hated in a garment. But I learned later that she wore the sweater, at least in part, because it smelled like me. Putting it on, she was able to ignore the knowledge we both had about my condition. She knew, however, that she was escorting me to a land she would have to explore on her own.

Other friends checked in. Ted and his wife, Jan, came up to see me. I had known them both for a half century. Pete and Katie, dear friends, visited, and my nephews and nieces, scattered all these years, emailed to tell me that they had heard of my diagnosis and they sent me hopes for my — what? My recovery? Hardly likely. But they wanted to say they loved me, and often did, and they wanted to relate the memories they held of me. I was charmed once when my niece Jennifer wrote to ask if the lion I had brought back from Africa was still alive behind the furnace in my father's old house. She had been a little girl when I returned from the Peace Corps, and I had made up a story about bringing back a lion. I had even suggested she go down in the basement to meet it, and in that wonderful conflu- ence of trust and doubt that small children exhibit, she had stalled on the top basement step, unsure whether to believe her uncle or her own skeptical understanding.

Now, decades later, she recalled the story, which meant, I realized, she recalled me as a young man.

Meanwhile, my story spread locally. I ran into a former colleague who seemed surprised to see me and exclaimed, "Man, you look good!"

As if he expected a difference. As if he had heard different.

Those types of interactions happened often. *You look good*, people said, their surprise, when weighed against their expectations, making them the tiniest bit rude. Susan said it was like being pregnant. Even people who knew better longed to reach out and touch a pregnant woman's stomach — and sometimes couldn't control themselves. Likewise, cancer invited people to offer opinions about my appearance. It seemed never to occur to them that they had overstepped; they would not have dreamed of saying that someone they met was obese or pale or suffering with bad skin. Cancer — and the concern around it — made them uninhibited.

They also sent prayers, something I hated. I knew they meant well, but I couldn't stand the arrogance of their position. First, they assumed I shared their belief to some degree or another. Second, they assumed if a god existed, then he or she was obviously a good and merciful god. I could have told them that a cursory reading of the Bible would have stood that concept on its head. The god of the Bible is a horrible, murderous creature, who creates a pre-Noah world, then destroys everything he just created, including innocent land animals, simply because he wasn't happy with the outcome of his project. He sends bears to kill children; he endorses slavery; he turns women to salt. Given his history, he's not a particularly good candidate to be an Emergency Contact person.

And finally, they failed to see the irony of their prayer. If an omniscient, omnipotent god wanted to help me out, then surely she or he could have prevented the entire thing from happening in the first place. Ditto, starving children and childhood leukemia while he's at it. As a result, I had to chew my tongue not to respond as I would have liked. Imagine if I had said to a parent who had lost a child that I would entreat Odin to let him or her go to Valhalla. They would have been insulted, but they could not imagine someone feeling equally insulted by their own superstitious wishes sent in my direction.

By and large, however, cancer unlocked the kindness in people. Whatever we had needed to fuss about, argue about, disagree about, suddenly became rather meaningless. It was true I was the one with cancer, not the other person, but they often had familiarity with the condition. I knew from reading that just shy of two million people experience cancer every year in the United States. Around six hundred thousand die. People knew cancer; they knew friends and family members who had suffered with it. If the topic came up in conversation, or if there was a reason for the person across from me to know about my circumstances, I always, always received kindness from them. At the same time — my son, Susan, my other family members and friends — all gave generously of themselves while receiving little in return. The attention was on me, not them, and in that way the equation felt out of balance. They would have to live with the pain of my absence, however that would fall on them. I would merely be gone.

I returned to my new normal life after the fishing trip, somewhat cautious and unsure of myself. Autumn moved in and began to pull the blanket up on another New England fall. Years before, I had planted a half dozen fruit trees in our yard, and this year, as it happened, was a bountiful harvest beyond any we had known. Justin, who had landed a teaching job in Concord, New Hampshire, developed a keen interest in the apples and pears and plums that grew in abundance outside our dooryard. Together with a wood shop class at his school, he designed and built a cider press, and soon we had fresh applesauce and cider when we liked. I enjoyed seeing him out among the trees, trees I had planted and loved, but I did not often join him. After the fishing trip, I had retired further into myself. I felt if not depression, at least a degree of futility that framed my daily life. I napped most middays, long, deep naps that brought me to the afternoon with little accomplished. Then again, I wondered what I was supposed to accomplish and whether the naps were a product of boredom or my medical condition. I withdrew a book from my agents' representation, finding it too trivial to continue on that particular story, then started a serious, intense novel about an old man on a shoreline in northern Quebec. I was writing about myself, of course, but I didn't care. Most days I went out to my small writing cabin and wrote what I could. I felt at sea, a little lost in my own world. Much of my writing career had been fueled by ambition, I realized, by the desire to hang what I had written on the refrigerator at home. Now I no longer cared what my sales figures might be, or whether a book had sufficient reach for a new market. The idea of trying to map my circumstances with a New York marketplace, to share a worldview with people ready for the latest thing, seemed grimly surreal. Even ads on TV seemed somewhat insane. The idea of a new soap, a new deodorant, a special slice of pizza, struck me as nearly insulting. Why in the world did we subject ourselves to such idiocy? And how was I to match whatever it was I wrote in my cabin to the American landscape of buy, sell, dispose? As Wordsworth had written, *The world is too much with us / getting and spending we lay waste our power.*

But if not spend myself in the pursuit of literature, of writing, well, then what would occupy me day to day?

I waited, but I was unsure of what I was waiting for. I watched Susan's reaction to see if she spotted anything to be concerned about in my lassitude. Occasionally I invented chores or errands for myself. Ironically, while cancer had made me concerned about time, how much of it I had left and so forth, now I found I had entire days with nothing to occupy me. An overabundance. I busied myself tidying up the house or straightening out old files — I spent most of one day deleting former student papers from my computer — and I tossed away tax returns older than five years. I also made an appointment with a lawyer and firmed up the details about my will. I elected my son as executor, checked off a Do Not Resuscitate option in my health contract, selected cremation for my remains, left the cottage in Maine to Susan, and signed over the rights to my literary output to Justin. Whatever I had been, however I would be remembered, struck me as nearly impossible to predict.

"So you want to be cremated?" Susan asked one day, trying to clarify.

"I guess so."

"I want to make sure whatever you want is carried out."

"Cremated, then, I guess."

"Okay, we'll do that."

I also discussed with a friend in Vermont the possibility of getting a drug that would cancel my life if I ended up confined to a bed. Vermont permits death-with-dignity and all I needed, from what we deduced, was a Vermont driver's license. My friend is a well-connected fellow, whose own father opted for euthanasia when his time came. He did not foresee any obstacle in getting a lethal cocktail prescribed by a colleague of his if that was the direction I wanted to take. He thought it would give me peace of mind to know death would come if I beckoned it, and I agreed. But we did not nail down who would administer the final drug or where I needed to be to carry out my wish without getting any friend or family member in trouble. Again, what had once been a theoretical question, one you could debate with impunity because it was not actually confronting you, now seemed decidedly real and powerful.

It all felt a little like planning a party you would not attend yourself. It also colored the shape and length of my days. How was I to resume some form of everyday life if simultaneously I needed to take steps to bring about my peaceful death? Still, I didn't want to be any more of a burden than I was already, so I moved forward on the necessary steps, not quite believing that the details mattered.

At about this time, I traveled to the New Hampshire seacoast to stay at Susan's for a weekend. Our houses are an hour and a half apart — I'm in the White Mountains and she is near the sea — and by the time I arrived in North Hampton my right leg had swollen and my ankle had tripled in size. Climbing out of the car, I felt astonished that my body could rebel over such a small exertion. I was merely driving, I told Susan. The swelling had come on all at once.

It was Saturday morning, but Susan insisted I call Dr. Dragnev's office. I hemmed and hawed for a half hour, then finally surrendered. Dr. Dragnev was not there when I finally gave in, but the doctor on call agreed with Susan's recommendation: I should go to the emergency room in Portsmouth and see what was happening in my body. Thirty minutes later, we were standing at a small desk in a construction zone — the hospital emergency entrance was under construction — giving my medical information, plus my insurance cards, to a lively young doctor who appeared to have his hands full.

"Just take a seat and we'll call you," he said after inducting me and arranging for a sonogram on my leg. "Shouldn't be too long."

They were concerned about blood clots. After getting another procedure done in a purposely dim room — a lubricated wand to bounce echoes off my soft tissue, if I understood it correctly — they led us to a gurney in the middle of a busy hallway and apologized that they did not have a room for us. Instead, they told us to sit, that the doctor would be along to go over the results, and that they were sorry again that no rooms were available. We sat. One of the things I treasure most about being with Susan is our ability to talk, to gab, to tell jokes and fill time. Often we will go an entire weekend, except when we are sleeping, simply talking and laughing without bothering to turn on a movie or radio. Being told to sit on a gurney in a busy hospital was no chore at all, except that we gradually grew aware of a young woman in a room directly across the hallway from us. She was being monitored by an LNA, a young man sitting in the hallway with a laptop, and we gradually realized that the young woman was a danger to herself. Twice while we watched she was visited by what we took to be a boyfriend and an older man who must have been her father. She possessed a nervous energy, not a healthy one, that seemed to send people away. We all know people like this: people who, though not in any way cruel or mean, somehow manage to be off-putting. The greater the need, the more people shy away. We even heard the boyfriend say he had a tee time, he couldn't stay, and the father insisted on getting her order right for take-out food. I tried to clear myself of all judgment, but I couldn't help wondering about this young woman, prepared to take her life, while I would have done anything to have my life, my full, active life, returned to me. I wanted to sneak into her room and tell her it would be all right, but of course I was being nosy and slightly insensitive. If illness taught me anything, it was that the things we think we know about other people are usually wrong or shortsighted. She was in profound pain, and the pain had caused her to try to harm herself. Many times while watching her, I hoped the boyfriend or father would simply shut up and take her in his arms and tell her he loved her.

Eventually a doctor came for me. She was a tall, young woman, who gladly took my phone and examined my Dartmouth patient portal to make sure she understood all the details.

"You have a clot behind your right knee," she said. "And that can be extremely dangerous. The clot could go to your heart or lung. We want to put you on blood thinners."

Standing beside us, she called Dr. Dragnev's office, had a brief consultation, then hung up and smiled at us.

"Once you're on the pills you'll be fine," she said. "Take ten milligrams, five in the morning, five in the evening. Don't wait on it. I'll put in the prescription right away."

"Thank you."

"Good luck with everything."

We hopped down off the gurney. While we had been talking to the doctor, the father of the young woman had departed, maybe to get food, maybe to keep an appointment he couldn't afford to miss. The young woman sat leaning against her boyfriend, obviously pleading for affection, while the boyfriend sat tightly against the wall, his nose buried in his phone, the warmth she required lost somewhere in the air around them.

One of the things I had hoped to do in retirement, a trip I hoped to take, was a March foray to Nebraska to see the migration of the sandhill cranes. I love animals. I had traveled to Yellowstone a half dozen times and I had always counted the visits — for fishing and for sightseeing — as highlights for any year. The proposed trip seemed fairly uncomplicated. Two days out, two days back, a few days watching the cranes along Nebraska's Platte River. Susan liked the sound of the trip, and I spent hours researching the right time to go, the best lodging opportunities, and so on. I sent Susan updates and reminded her, more than once, that no less a conservationist than Jane Goodall had pronounced that the migration of the sandhill cranes was one of the great animal migrations on earth. She recommended it.

Thinking about the cranes and the trip, however, I began to question whether, at some level, it would not be better to continue into the wild, as it were, and end my life privately. Understand: This was not a product of depression or anger. I had a clear understanding for how I could live and die for the next few months or years. I knew that Justin and Susan would do everything they could to make my final days comfortable and worthwhile. But part of me, my Odysseus mind, wondered if I shouldn't select my own time and place, my own ending, and relieve them of the burden of the many delicate decisions and compromises they would be forced to make as death approached. Frankly, I wondered if it was not politer to take care of this last business in a clean, uncomplicated way. Why subject my loved ones, and myself, to the various indignities of invalidhood? Would it be commendable, and somehow truer to my nature, to find a way to secret my body and finish things as my sickness demanded? I had never been particularly dependent on any other human. Why permit myself that invidious luxury now? Marcus Aurelius had informed me for years that we only live in a single day; that to live shorter than our expectation is no great injustice. He reminds his readers often that oblivion, and therein peace, is a mere dagger away.

I didn't tell Susan any hint of this, although she knew I entertained thoughts about death by my own hand. I wasn't sure, honestly, how serious I was about it. At the beginning of my illness, she had asked that I promise her I wouldn't simply disappear. She said she needed to make sure she could say goodbye to me, and I had given her my word. Besides, when one thought seriously about ways to end life, the plans did not seem simple. I went through various scenarios, toying with ideas, discarding each when it struck me as too cruel to the person who might recover my body, or too mystifying to Justin and Susan. I also worried that I might botch the job — as many unfortunately do — and manage somehow to wound myself grievously, but not fatally.

Gloomy thoughts, perhaps. I knew that suicidal ideation is an alarm bell in the mental health community, but I did not feel in the least drawn to death. I felt, instead, a desire to relieve those around me of a difficult burden. I also reserved for myself the right to call an end to my life. In the final analysis, I told myself to wait, to observe, but not to kid myself about the state of my health. It was possible I had years, not months, and I planned to use them as well as I could.

That's where things stood when my oldest brother, Bill, contacted me and asked if he could come to visit. He was plain about it. He said he didn't put much stock in going to funerals, but visiting someone before she or he died — that made sense to him.

Because I had grown up in New Jersey, however, and because Bill was driving up with his son, Stephen, from Virginia, I suggested I meet him in our old hometown of Westfield. I had several reasons for proposing the trip. I didn't want Bill, who is eighty-four, to drive all the way from Virginia to New Hampshire simply to say hello. He is in good health, and has resources to afford such a journey, but I realized a trip to New Jersey on my part would save him some travel and would also give me the opportunity to visit my two sisters, Joanie and Cathy. It also happened to be the fiftieth anniversary of my high school class, the 1971 graduating Blue Devils of Westfield High School. Covid concerns had canceled a class reunion scheduled for the fall, but it left me with an itch to see my boyhood home, to prove my memory against the reality of those early years, and I made dates with various family members to visit them over the long weekend before Thanksgiving. Susan wasn't able to shake out of work, and neither was Justin, so I went on my own, driving the familiar path to my hometown down the Merritt and Garden State Parkways.

Before seeing anyone, in a little window of time I had built deliberately into the trip, I decided to visit my childhood neighborhood, a few streets that wound through a portion of Westfield that had been my playground. The weather was good; the sun hit the streets and land in the way I remembered. I parked in front of my house, a modest, but solid two-story home, a place where I had lived with my parents, Charles and Deborah, where I had slept contentedly in the heart of a large, Irish Catholic family. Here was where my mother and father died, where John recovered from a motor scooter accident, where Cathy announced her engagement, where Joanie, bravely bucking moribund tradition, declared that she, a young woman, wanted to go to college. Here was where my brother Mike climbed on the den roof and jumped down to the bushes in a daring late-night escape, and where once it had rained so hard, then froze, that we could skate on the driveway while our parents watched from a picture window. Here was where Chuck, Charles Jr., came home from the University of Maryland, where he swam on the college team, his late-evening arrivals on Christmas Eve as exciting as Santa's. Here were Easter ducks and Christmas Ping-Pong, birthday candles on Duncan Hines cakes, and Wiffle Ball games in the backyard, two squares of the garage door a perfect strike zone.

Here was Ben Cartwright, and Samantha Stephens, Paladin, Cheyenne, *Mission: Impossible, The Wonderful World of Disney, Peyton Place,* the Yankees, the New York Giants; here was Cousin Brucie playing the Top 40 on AM radio and, coincidentally, the soundtrack of our days, and later, Alison Steele the Nightbird, host of an early FM station out of New York City, her voice a cool guide to someplace we wanted to discover but could hardly fathom at that point; here was *Lad: A Dog, Call of the Wild, Ivanhoe,* the Hardy Boys, *The Kid Who Batted 1.000, Stuart Little, Charlotte's Web,* and even, in high school, the misty mountains of Tolkien's dream. Here were spaghetti dinners, turkeys, barbecued chicken with our own special sauce, vodka and rye, Pabst Blue Ribbons, Porky my childhood beagle, and the rosebushes that stood no chance against seven growing children.

Just a house. Just my house. Unexceptional in all ways except for the lives that existed there for a time, moved on, died, married, had children. Just a house that could still hold the sound of my mother calling up the stairs, *Bill, Chuck, John, Cathy, Joanie, Mike, and Joe . . . come to dinner. Time for church. Close the windows, rain is coming.*

Up the street, where I played daily with Monte and Brad and Dougie and Timmy and Missy and Jane, and Margret Van Deussen (her name was always said in a rush, all three names colliding together), all childhood friends, I stood for a long time and studied the two trees that served as the base for all of our operations. They were two black gum trees, or pricker ball trees as we knew them, with a perfect scaffolding of branches that allowed us access. We were good climbers, all of us, and once we left the ground we performed as perfect little apes, jumping — dangerously, honestly — from branch to branch, finding little notches where we could lounge in comfort, able, when a car passed by, to lob a fistful of pricker balls — brown, gnarly little seedcases — at it. We spent entire afternoons in those trees, chattering and happy, and standing beside them now, the lowest branches pruned away so that a mower could swing his machine below it, I felt tearful and grateful for the little boys and girls who had played out their early life there. I did not, however, achieve a grand reckoning. If anything, I felt a wistful haze, a dream state where I could remember, imperfectly, the feel of the tree's bark on my bare hand, the smell of green grass, the summer languor of draping ourselves on the tree's branches and feeling power in our invisibility.

Afterward, I drove around Westfield, retraced familiar routes. The town, a well-heeled New York suburb, still looked much the same as it had as I grew up. I stopped at the high school football field and walked around the small stadium. I had played high school football there, baseball, too, and what I recalled in that moment was a single day during that long-ago summer before our senior year when my health had been so robust, so unquestioned, that I ran through the entire town merely for the joy of feeling my body move. The running boom had just taken hold thanks to Jim Fixx and others, and to run a mile seemed like a remarkable thing, but on that day I ran five or six miles easily, gliding on the cement walkways, jumping over small obstacles whenever I came to one, acknowledging the occasional high school honk of friends spotting me and saying hello. Now, standing on the fifty-yard line of our great triumphs — we went undefeated our senior year and won the state championship — I realized that I was a silly old man, cancerous, nostalgic, hoping that to feel the past was to regain the past, while knowing, without question, that some part of me lived here among my teammates, lived in the earnest work we had done together, but that it was gone, meaningless to anyone who had not stepped onto this field a half century before as a boy striving to be a man.

I knew, too, that I would not be back to this town. All of this, all of the trip, had been an excuse to come and say goodbye. I had lived in New Hampshire far longer than I had lived here, but one is given only a single childhood, and mine had been spent here among the sprinklers and edged sidewalks, the careful hedges and gleaming lights of well-appointed living rooms. Westfield, New Jersey, had launched me — despite my eventual mistrust of its corporate values, its Republican base and wealth — and sent me away from it, first to Philadelphia for college, then to Africa in the Peace Corps, and then on and on through young adulthood, loss, joy, to streams and wild rivers, canoe trips, mountain hikes, camping trips in the glaciers of Wyoming, into small cabins beside lakes and onto the runners of a dogsled behind our beloved animals pulling through a New Hampshire winter.

*Anemoia* is an arcane word used to express nostalgia for a time we never experienced; it describes the feeling we have, regardless of our upbringing, for the allure and inviting loneliness of a train whistle heard from great distance. But standing on that football field, then walking slowly to my car where I would drive to see my brother and sisters, I felt nostalgia not for a land I had never experienced, but for my own youthful life, and for the great goodness of my family and the care and tenderness of a community that had sheltered and nurtured me without ever asking whether I needed it or not.

# 7

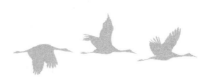

In time I discovered some strange, but intriguing, consolations in having a terminal diagnosis. For example, I realized, after I had returned to New Hampshire, that I would never need to buy another piece of clothing. Not one thing. No suitcoat, no dress shoes, no new sneakers. I didn't need another bottle of cologne. All of my appliances, washing machines, vacuums, even my current automobile, were sufficient. They would last me until I no longer needed them. As a result, many of the usual pressing concerns of daily life faded away. Suddenly little in my world seemed to be "my problem."

Should I paint the house this year? Not my problem.

Repair the broken window on the porch? Not my problem.

Order more cordwood, increase the piping diameter in the basement sink, plant a hedge, fix a fence? Not my problem.

Initially, at least, the new realization that time, in this one small way, favored me, brought me a tinge of welcome wickedness in my thinking.

Moreover, the money I had carefully saved for retirement, hoping, as I did, to shepherd it through twenty years of simplified living, now seemed an outsized pool of money that I would not, could not, spend or substantially dent in the time remaining to me. A good problem to have, of course, but how odd, near the end, to realize much of what I spent my life collecting no longer seemed important, or properly sized, in the least. My son, Justin, told me I should take a trip to Thailand, blow a part of the money on a fancy camper and pickup, go spend the winter in a condo someplace warm. Because of the brevity of the time left to me, I was suddenly wealthier — relatively — than I had ever imagined.

He also told me I should get a dog.

"You love dogs," he said, which of course was true. "And maybe this time the dog would outlive you. That's a nice twist on an old story."

That sense of economy, of conserving something that no longer needed conserving, spilled over into other aspects of my daily life. Without any thought, I could delete hundreds of emails and contacts from my computer. If I no longer needed a new sweater, neither did I need a fresh invitation to bargains on shopping sites, or offers of loans from a local credit union. The world of commerce, the spinning carousel of reaching for a prize, no longer touched me. Cancer, I grudgingly admitted, had given me a useful filter, so much so that I found dealing with social contacts became elementary. For one thing, I had the world's greatest excuse to slip out of any obligation; I possessed the ultimate trump card, the best get-out-of-jail-free card of all time. Not only would a potential host excuse me, but she or he would offer commiseration that I didn't feel up to doing X or Y. For a person with a reclusive lean to his personality, I had gained an unqualified freedom.

But despite all these curious benefits, I couldn't shake the reality that I had to drain my lung every other day and record the measure and hue of discharge. No get-out-of-jail-free card proved effective on that central fact. In late fall, thinking I should put the old post office in Maine to bed for the winter, I traveled up to Pembroke by myself. On a certain late evening, I sat at the small table where Susan and I had held the phone consultation after first receiving the diagnosis. In the quiet light of the Chubby coal stove, my eyes fixed on the water outside, I stripped off my shirt and walked my way through the procedure of draining my chest. I had performed the operation a couple of times on my own, but I didn't like to do so. I particularly didn't like looking at the small slit in my chest, a red, lipless mouth, the incision into which the catheter tube slithered down to my lung. It felt as if I had entered a vintage black-and-white movie, a scene in which a lost, forlorn man confronts himself in a mirror and finds he is disgusted by the vision returned to him. The feeling of health, the gain I had made with Tagrisso, seemed illusory. I couldn't kid myself that things were improving if I had to wipe down my chest with alcohol pads, wear protective gloves so that I didn't infect the incision, adjust the dial on the pressurized bottles to draw sufficiently, but not too hard, so that the small sea around my lung might relinquish its hold on the expansion of my breath. In that dim light, I had to watch the liquid transfer to the bottle, wondering whether I had yielded enough, if more would possibly help my long-term prospects, if I had somehow contaminated myself inadvertently. Then, afterward, I had to bandage my chest with a dura-patch, an intensely adhesive bandage that glued itself to my skin and pressed the serpentine coils of plastic tubing against my heart.

When I finished, and after I had put the medical equipment out of sight, I poured myself a scotch and carried the glass out onto the small deck overlooking the water. The stars had already appeared; Saturn or Venus — I could never remember which was which — hovered just above the southern horizon. I sipped my drink and studied the sky. *How did this end?* I wondered. I worried if I was being naive, that, in every real sense, it was already over. I feared being the prototypical soldier, wounded grievously on the battlefield, who looks up to his comrade and asks if it is bad. I considered that I might be missing the vital understanding I required to navigate these last months, years, days with appropriate aplomb. It was possible that others — however kindly intended — already saw death on me. Several times in my life I had encountered people with cancer, and I knew it was possible to see it and know it before the afflicted person recognized it in her- or himself. My own mother had not known, fully, the severity of her diagnosis. That had been approved medical protocol in those days. It struck me as a hideous practice now, but it was customary then to lie to patients, tell them less than they needed to know, allow them to live in the delusional promise of returning health. Eventually, naturally, the illness would claim them, but it was part of a poorly conceived system to keep them in the dark as much as possible. The casual cruelty of that approach, the unrealized arrogance of the care-takers, seemed incomprehensible by modern standards. And yet maybe, in kindness, Susan and Justin — and perhaps the medical team — downplayed the critical nature of my diagnosis in order to lend me hope.

I didn't like the thought of that. Standing on the deck looking out, the lovely burn of scotch now and then on the roof of my mouth, I wondered how I would know when the cancer had won. That day would come, I knew, and it concerned me that I might be too dim, too confused, to know the battle had ended. I wanted to preserve what dignity I could, to reserve for myself the best path for my ending. I imagined the palliative team would speak honestly to me; that was a large part of its purpose, as I understood it. Nevertheless, that didn't help necessarily when I walked into a room of people who knew my diagnosis and I saw them weighing my condition with their eyes. Cancer patients live in danger of becoming the cancer, the grasping disease, their previous identity surrendered and replaced with the newer, more dynamic character of a dying person, a host to the tiger inside them.

My weight began to climb back. I had been 183 before Tagrisso, and now, months after I commenced the regimen, I began to put on weight. I soon passed 190 and hovered for a time at 194. It felt good. Susan, seeing me begin to fill out, confessed that she had been alarmed by my rapid weight loss earlier in the year. In fact, she said, she had been fairly certain that I was on my way out merely from the dimension of my waistline and the gauntness in my face.

"You went through entire days and ate nothing but apple-sauce or yogurt," she reminded me. "Justin and I both watched you like hawks to see what you were eating."

"I wasn't hungry then."

"Well, I'm always glad to see you eat."

With the increase in weight, an interesting reversal in my lungs began occurring. At last, the sea of pleural effusion began to subside. Where I had been yielding nine hundred milliliters in the early summer (and two thousand milliliters the first time with Dr. Backer), the output began to diminish. I knew, from discussions with Dr. Dragnev and Dr. Backer, that the level of pleural effusion would dictate when, and if, I could remove the catheter from my lung. If I reached a steady level, somewhere south of a hundred milliliters, it could come out. In fact, Dr. Backer suggested that consistent draining, done every day, would be the fastest path to removal of the catheter. He recommended it and encouraged me to be hopeful about it.

For the first time in this long summer and fall, I said no. No to the recommendations. No to draining every day. Justin said I was being hardheaded, but the truth, honestly, was that the sight of the drain, the choreography of draining my lung, the amber glaze of the liquid — like chicken broth, one of us quipped on a summer night — filled me with despair. At times when I was engaged in some activity, or having fun of some kind, I could forget the catheter and, to a limited degree, forget my illness momentarily. It was never completely gone from my mind, of course, but it could retreat or sink temporarily into the buzz of a pleasant occupation. On the other hand, stripping off my shirt nightly, pulling the dura-patch bandage off my chest (carefully so as not to pull a cord attached to my lung), putting on gloves and then washing everything with alcohol wipes, attaching the bottle to the line in my chest, wedging it below me so that I wouldn't have to see it, talking cheerily while the hole in my chest led directly to my lung, feeling the odd, pawing sensation in my chest cavity as the lung began to re-expand along the shoreline of retreating effusion, then waiting, still chatting, maybe watching the news until finally the drip of liquid slowed and became nearly incidental, reminded me that I was a sick, weary old man whose lungs could not demand or conquer the space nature had allotted to them.

Draining every day, I would be conscious of being sick every day. I couldn't bear that thought.

I waited and I watched. On several draining days, the liquid hardly appeared at all. Justin again urged me to drain every day, assuring me that that approach had the best chance of success. He was correct, I knew, and so was Dr. Backer, but I simply couldn't do it.

Around this time, the principal of the Warren elementary school — our local school whose playground abutted my property — called and asked if I would be willing to come in and discuss one of my young adult books, *Game Change*, if the current sixth-grade class agreed to read it and generate questions. I had done this kind of thing many times before, for adult and school groups alike, but months had gone by since I had spoken publicly about anything at all. I felt rusty and unsure of my breathing, though a part of me — a part I suspected Susan would endorse — thought I needed to have something on my calendar besides medical appointments. After I had agreed tentatively to the date, the teacher of the class, a young woman in her first year named Abby Arsenault, wrote me a note and thanked me for agreeing to speak, and then she requested I come up with questions I wanted to ask them about the book. It was a nice twist on the usual presentation format. It made me feel more comfortable — I was not the whole show, but merely an author being interviewed — and I said I looked forward to doing it. I also told her I had lung cancer, and she reassured me that my little local elementary school had a full mask mandate.

It was a small event, obviously, but I inflated it with more importance than I would have under normal circumstances. It astonished me to discover, the night before the event, that I had forgotten which clothes I typically wore to give a talk or even to teach a class. I had also put on the back shelf of my mind my well-rehearsed introductions about writing, books, and the importance of reading. I was rusty, in other words. After teaching for three decades, I felt nervous about speaking to a handful of sixth graders. To make it a little more complex, I debated about the advisability of walking to the meeting. It was ridiculously close, just the next building over from my house more or less, but I didn't know how certain I could be of my breath. I didn't want to arrive entirely out of air, wheezing and gasping, while the sixth graders wondered what kind of speaker had been unleashed on them. To drive over, however, seemed the worst kind of concession to make to the cancer.

I decided to chance it. I walked to the school, dressed in what I had finally recalled to be my teaching clothes, and rang through to the principal's office. It took me a moment outside the door to ease my breathing. Michael Galli, principal, fellow writer, and sometime chicken farmer, came to the door and invited me inside. He had good energy, as the saying goes. He obviously liked schools, liked being among children trying to make their way, and so did I. When we walked down a short hallway to the classroom where the sixth graders had collected, he said hello to a bunch of kids, each one acknowledging his greeting with a smile and a shy reply.

At the appropriate moment, we stepped into the classroom. Even the short walk down the hallway, unfortunately, had winded me. I smiled and introduced myself to Abby; she was young and entirely in tune with her class. She had arranged the desk chairs so that I would be seated in front of a semicircle of students, all of them sitting with my book in front of them, their attention miraculously pointed at me.

Slowly, as if opening up an old attic trunk, I introduced myself. I still had difficulty breathing; I had to cough several times, trying to get my airway unclogged. Then, gradually, much to my relief, I began to remember how I had done this thing for so many years. Though they didn't know it, they had been much in my mind when I wrote *Game Change*. On the face of it, it is a conventional story about a high school senior, a second-string quarterback behind an All-State superstar, who is suddenly propelled into starting the state championship game when the superstar blows out his knee. The football game was the bait, as I conceived it, to get a student's interest in the narrative.

The main character, Zeb, however, was not so conventional, I hoped. He was derived from my imagination, true, but he was the product of the rural segment of New Hampshire, the segment to which these students belonged, who did not have easy lives. Zeb resides with his mother in a poorly insulated

Shasta camper plugged into his uncle Pushee's home. His father is gone; his mother works at a diner — where she will not be able to take a day off to watch him in the championship game — and collects Hummel statuettes she can ill afford from thrift stores. In short, the book was about them, about these students collected in this economically strained community, and I wondered, nervously, if they would be offended or find something useful in the story. Rural poverty has been an abiding issue in my young adult novels — New Hampshire rural poverty — and I was genuinely curious to gauge their reactions.

They liked it, or at least said they did. Gradually I became aware of the fine teaching, the excellent prep work, Abby had done with the class. Not only had they read the book, and discussed it, they had also "mapped" some of the characters, charting their words or innermost thoughts, on a drawing they made themselves. They were prepared; they were keen to discuss the themes of the novel, and I remembered, as we dove into it, feeling the wonder and satisfaction of teaching — feelings I had missed without recognizing it. Here we were on a midweek morning discussing what it means to be poor, what it means to feel unsure of your meals or your electricity, what opportunity signifies, how do you navigate friends and relatives, what does free enterprise do to the losers in the system, how does a parent's departure affect the remaining family, what is society's responsibility to those individuals having a difficult time surviving?

It was as good and as rich a discussion as I had ever experienced in a classroom. And I felt, halfway through it, incredibly grateful that these students had given their frankness so freely. As an author, I was pleased to know that what I thought was in the novel was indeed there, ready to be absorbed by anyone who cared to read it.

Afterward we talked about books and reading and which novels they liked. They recommended a dozen books I didn't know, but I wrote them down and made a note to order them. Little by little, the distance between a visiting speaker and the class members broke down into a chatty session. We were readers; we were citizens of New Hampshire in all that that meant.

Everyone contributed except one boy sitting on the right of the half circle.

Afterward, after posing for a picture with the group for the local newsletter, after looking at the character maps they had produced — and even laminating them! — after talking with one boy about sharks (we were/are both shark fanatics, and I had brought them a novel I had written for Scholastic about a shark detective, one he had already claimed for his own), after thanking Abby for the superb job she did in prepping them, I walked back down the hallway with Michael. He said he thought it had gone great, as I did, but when I brought up the one boy in the class who didn't speak, he stopped and looked at me.

"He lives in circumstances similar to Zeb," he said in a whisper. "I wondered how he would react to it. It was my only worry in this whole visit."

"Zeb probably wouldn't read a book about his own life, would he?"

Michael shook his head. Then I was outside again, walking home, my breath still labored. I felt strangely moved by the entire experience, rewarded and wistful, reminded in the best way what literature, what reading, could carry into a room. I was a teacher, when all was said and done. The cancer had made me forget that, and I vowed to not let it rob me in that particular way ever again.

After two weeks of low drainage flows, after one or two sessions when my lung yielded nothing at all, Dr. Backer agreed to remove the catheter from my chest. It was the best news I had

had in months. It indicated a half dozen benchmarks of improvement: The pleural effusion was slower to build, the Tagrisso worked as predicted, the cancer cells throughout my body had been reduced by the medication. It was a good day when I got the okay to make an appointment. I scheduled it for a Friday and planned to go alone. Susan and Justin had to work, and Dr. Backer assured me it was a brief, painless removal.

"I hate for you to go alone," Susan told me the night before on the phone. "It's such a lonely thing to do."

"It will be all right. It shouldn't take very long at all."

"Still, I hate it."

She could not be at every medical appointment no matter how hard she tried. Neither could Justin. It was implied in our conversation around the appointment, not overtly stated, that it was wiser to bank the release time from work for the inevitable day when I would truly need them by my side. Besides, by this time, I was something of a veteran at Dartmouth-Hitchcock, so the prospect of a solo visit did not concern me. I knew where to park, how to arrange my visit, when the new pizza came out of the ovens in the centrally located snack bar. I knew how early to report ahead of an appointment, what sorts of shoes to wear (slide on and off), whether I would need to eat a chalk-based disk before receiving my bone-health injection, and what kind of book made sense to have on hand for reading. Given the featurelessness of my calendar, I did not mind the casual pace of a day at Dartmouth.

When the time came for my removal appointment — after going off blood thinners for three days — I was escorted to the same room where Dr. Backer had first explained my diagnosis and then drained me. As before, I worked with the LNA to record my medical numbers. The LNA was a pleasant young woman who asked me — as Dartmouth policy required — to give my name and birthdate at least three times during our brief meeting. It amused us both. Then she left and Dr. Backer arrived with a student doctor in tow, a young woman who looked to be about thirty. Dartmouth is a teaching hospital, I knew, but this was the first time in my cancer journey that any student had joined one of my doctors. She introduced herself and I answered back, but, due to Covid, we did not shake hands.

Dr. Backer processed the requisite paperwork at the small desk in the corner of the room. He asked how I felt. I told him I felt great. At this point I would have said anything to get the catheter removed, but I also grew aware that once the catheter came out, I would no longer be able to remove the pleural effusion if it caused me trouble. It felt as if we were about to do something final. I knew, intellectually, that we could likely replace the catheter in a day or two if my condition deteriorated, but psychologically the stakes seemed higher. To reinsert the catheter would be a signpost of my approach to death. It would mean that whatever had worked to free me of the hole in my lung and the attached rubber tubing had at last begun to fail.

The removal was less than dramatic. I lay back on the examination table, shirtless, while Dr. Backer explained what needed to occur. He spoke to me as much as to the student doctor. He mentioned that it could conceivably cause me some pain or discomfort and that — although highly unlikely — the point of the buried needle could break off in my chest. The sound of that, the image of that, chilled me, and I said as much to Dr. Backer. He reassured me that it was quite rare to have anything of the sort happen, but I recalled that I had signed a document stipulating that I understood the risks involved. Legal coverage, of course. I wondered, absently, how you would get a catheter removed if you did not agree to sign the acknowledgment. I also wondered how a doctor would go about retrieving the recalcitrant needle if it had, in fact, become lodged in my chest.

As it happened, Dr. Backer was an excellent teacher. He permitted the student doctor to perform the extraction, but I was keenly aware of his face hovering above her shoulder. He spoke calmly and succinctly. He kept his attention intensely focused. It may have been a routine procedure, I realized, but he was responsible for withdrawing the business end of a needle from my lung. For a long moment, I stared up at two faces, four eyes, focused on the delicate procedure. Then, with no discomfort whatsoever, Dr. Backer said I was all set.

"It's out?" I asked, hardly believing that such a central part of my illness had been removed so calmly.

"It's out," he said.

I remained on the table for a few minutes to make sure my wound would not bleed. Afterward, Dr. Backer bandaged me, explaining as he did so that I needed to keep the incision area clean, that I should still keep it covered in the shower for the time being, and that, despite my hopes to swim this late in the season, I needed to stay out of the water for at least ten days or until the wound was properly closed.

"Thank you," I said to Dr. Backer when I sat up again.

It seemed an underwhelming expression of gratitude. Here was a man who had supervised the draining of my lung, who had inserted a catheter into my chest and removed it, who had explained, delicately, the reality of my diagnosis. He had performed every action, every conversation, with flawless skill. He had taken every pain to preserve my humanity, to be as gentle as possible in his depiction of what was going on inside my body, and now, things go as they might, we had probably come to the end of our association.

"Keep doing what you're doing," I said.

What I meant was that I valued his work. That I valued his kindness. That I had a glimpse of the vast knowledge base from which he drew. Fissured through our communication, I had seen his dedication and expertise, his compassion for the patients under his care. And I imagined that as a young doctor he would give aid and comfort to thousands of patients for many years to come. His work was brilliant, and I wanted him, somehow, to know I appreciated it.

*It's out,* I texted Susan as soon as I left the hospital.

*Did it hurt?*

*Not at all.*

I drove home slowly, passing through the glorious autumn landscape. I drove beside the Connecticut River and looked out to see if I could spot the Dartmouth crew team. They often practiced on the river, but I did not see them that day. I was more than halfway home when I realized I had been driving with my left hand, while my right hand stayed cupped over the bandage on my chest, as if, I realized, I could not be certain of my good fortune.

Susan had worked many years among the New Hampshire disability community — her first teaching job was in a "special ed" program — and she had made me attuned to the language bias implicit in many of society's discussions around that subject. Perhaps her biggest contribution to my own unschooled vocabulary was the placement of the disability before the name of the individual. Blind John Thomas, rather than John Thomas, who happens to be blind. It sounds simple and easily fixed, but the importance of keeping the human in front of the disability was critical. A human was not the disability; she or he was human first and a person with a certain condition afterward.

My cancer diagnosis, I realized, threatened to ignite a similarly troublesome conversation in my own mind. Was I Cancer Patient Mr. X, or Mr. X who had a cancer diagnosis? It seemed important to rank the cancer diagnosis in second place, squarely below markers of my personal identification. Cancer, and all the attendant preoccupation of pills, appointments, CT scans, X-rays, bone medications, and so forth, could rapidly become my self-conception. I did not want to become a parody of myself, a bearded old man whose main claim for attention was his illness. It was tempting, and potentially spirit-killing, to give myself over to an identity as a sick person rather than as a healthy person.

The removal of the catheter had gone miles to bring me back to myself, but I was still incapable of physical exertion. Cutting the lawn one last time in the fall, I had to stop after every swath to rest and catch my breath. I wasn't certain if I should push myself through — an old athlete's reflex — or refrain from pushing too hard. Carrying groceries to the car, climbing stairs with a messenger bag over my shoulder, sweeping the porch with a push broom, forced me to stop frequently and pant like an old dog until I could continue. I knew from conversations with Melissa Storm, the nurse practitioner who was part of Dr. Dragnev's team, that moderate walking was heartily recommended. In fact, I had promised her that I would try to get into a regular walking regimen, primarily to keep my body strong, but understanding that intention did not make it easier to breathe when my lung failed to provide me with air. The man I had been a minute before the diagnosis would have pushed through any amount of discomfort for a greater gain of physical health; the cancer patient I had become had first to accommodate the illness, then consider the performance of my body.

Susan and I traveled to Maine one last time before the weather made visits more ordeal than pleasure. It was cold when we arrived and I hurried to make a coal fire in our stove. The sun now set sooner; the leaves on the aspens near the water edge had already abandoned most of their holds on the trees. The water appeared cold and gray, a pewter that approaching winter seemed to draw up from the bottom of the estuary. Gulls remained on the mud banks at low tide, but many of the birds we had enjoyed through the summer had migrated. The great bald eagle that often landed on the tall pine overlooking the sea failed to appear. The little cottage seemed a soft light in an otherwise dark countryside.

We had come to swim. Or I had come to swim. The idea of going into the ocean, on a shore that we loved, seemed more important to me than I could say. This was where, in spring, I had accepted the diagnosis of cancer; it was here that I had told Susan what had happened and the idea of death had begun to seep into our lives. The world had changed for us here, and somehow by swimming, by a full immersion into the ocean we watched all summer, I hoped not to regain anything, really, but to announce to myself that I had returned at least for a little while to the life and retirement for which I had worked.

We had made our plans while consulting the weather, and so the next morning we were not surprised to find ourselves in a reasonably warm day for that late in the early-winter season. We had coffee on the deck overlooking the water, and it was tempting to remain beside the house, out of the wind, where we could get the benefit of the sun without the chill that would follow a swim. But I was determined to make an attempt. Bullheaded, maybe, but I felt I wanted to do something mildly reckless, something hale and hearty and far removed from Dartmouth-Hitchcock, from rubber tubes in my chest, from the fat horse pills I had to consume daily, from the probing glint of a hypodermic needle, from the knotted congestion of my reluctant left lung. It was silly, really, but I needed a benchmark, a place from which to navigate.

"You should go in naked!" Susan told me. "What are they going to do? Arrest you?"

"Maybe I will."

"Kind of mythic."

I didn't go naked, but standing above the waterline, staring out at the wedge of water stirred by the Reversing Falls of local fame, I paused and tried to hold true to my plan. We had been on this beach many times, to clam, to swim, to sun and walk. I was aware that maybe I was overdoing this whole thing. Maybe I was lending it more weight than it deserved. Honestly, to swim or not to swim made no difference whatsoever. I knew that, but still, after kissing Susan — who had made the sane decision not to swim — I tried to walk boldly into the softly stirring water and dunk down. Surprisingly, the water was not painfully cold, but I cannot say there was anything bold about the way I finally entered. I turned, looked at Susan, and then fell backward into a patch of water about waist-deep. No Australian crawl, no breathy breaststroke. I remained under for a three-count, struggled to get to my feet, then stood in the late-autumn air feeling more victorious than the small dunking warranted. It was cold, yes, but it felt vital and hungry and full of life. As it turned out, I hadn't been completely wrong about the impulse to go swimming. It gave me something, maybe a pyrrhic victory, but in the shadow of cancer I took what wins I could.

We went back to the cottage, and there I fell more in love with Susan.

I had loved her for a long time, close to eight years, but lately, since the illness had invaded our days, I had seen a Susan I had merely glimpsed before. Her kindness, and her deep understanding, had made me realize that nothing could come between us. A cliché, of course, but back in the cottage, the Chubby coal stove throwing fine heat, I looked at her and felt such an overwhelming mixture of love, admiration, trust, and gratitude that it stopped me. Had she always been standing there before me? I watched her move around our tiny cabin, her face almost always in a smile, and I wondered how it was that we so rarely saw someone all the way through. I could list a thousand things I admired about Susan, could talk at length about our adventures together, but had I ever taken the time, the true opportunity, to study this person who stood closer to me than anyone else? Maybe, I considered, true love — if it existed as the poets promised — was not the knee-weakening swell that fed young love. Maybe true love, instead, was the ability finally to see the person who shared your bed, your interests, your daily life. Maybe cancer, in its finality, provided me with the lens to see her all the way around. I knew what occupied her, what worried her, what delighted her. I knew her body and her tears, and I knew what she was like in the middle of the night when we often reached toward each other to confirm our own existence. Most of us know the opening lines of Elizabeth Barrett Browning's famous poem that begins with a question: *How do I love thee?* Then the assertion: *Let me count the ways.*

My love for Susan, however, rested in the later lines of the poem, the middle verses that explained how Browning's love was particular for her beloved.

> *I love thee to the level of every day's*
> *Most quiet need, by sun and candle-light.*

To every day's most quiet need. I felt my heart expand while watching her, felt immensely proud of her goodness — and that she lent it, to the degree she could, to me, to her daughters and parents, to her siblings and students. I realized that my heart's travel was finished; that it rested with her, would always be hers, until my last breath.

Christmas arrived with its usual demands and pleasures, the longest night of the year folded into the festive season. On Christmas morning, Susan and I remained in bed and watched the launch of the James Webb Telescope. We had been following the launch preparations casually, impressed by what we learned about its mission from Justin. He had been doing a unit on space exploration with his class, and he had shown them several NASA videos about the telescope, its design and function, then passed along the information to us. It was on our radar, so to speak, but it was Christmas and we had put it to one side while we shopped and prepared for the holidays. Perhaps, honestly, we were guilty, as many Americans seem to be, of treating space exploration as either so safe as to be no concern to us any longer, or so common as to be uninteresting. The James Webb, we knew, would not be set fully into orbit until well into the new year, after a million miles of voyaging, nor would it begin sending back data and photos until midsummer. Tuning in to what we imagined would be a routine launch might be easily skipped; it was scheduled for dawn, and in the cold winter months in New Hampshire, dawn brought a deep, hollow start to a day. Besides, the launch had been postponed once or twice already, and Christmas morning, with all its myth, did not seem a propitious time for science.

With coffee in bed, we checked on the launch and discovered that it had been reset for a reasonable hour, somewhere around 7:30 A.M., and that the coverage from the NASA website had a pregame lineup of interesting interviews with scientists who hoped to employ the Webb's capabilities in their own research. The telecast of the information, the format of the interviews, were decidedly no-nonsense; here was science, pure science, and it did not need the din of ads and products shouting for a spot in the marketplace that plagued everyday television. Amid all the political conflict of the past few years, immune to the perennial demands of the free enterprise system, the program seemed a beacon of what was good about our country, about the world, about the insatiable human desire for exploration and knowledge. When the countdown eventually commenced, Susan and I held hands and — ridiculously — I felt my eyes fill. Here, in its purity, was a good hope. When the range operation manager saw the telescope separate from its rocket carrier a few minutes later, when everything, everything had worked perfectly, he raised his hand and exhorted with a French accent, *Go Webb!*

Go to space. Go a million miles into the universe. Go to the edge of time and report back. Tell us, at last, who we are.

I don't believe in the power of prayer, but I recognize one when I see it. Thirty years of work, ten billion dollars of investment, ten thousand contributors, and everything worked more perfectly than anyone dared hope. This was the repudiation of the Tower of Babel; humans had come together from around the world and had cooperated on this magnificent project. I couldn't remember being so moved by something; I was inspired by the matter-of-fact atmosphere of the launch, by the international flavor of the event, and by the profound scientific inquiry lingering beneath the placid demeanor of the launch room.

When at last the gold-plated sunshield unfurled — an engineering feat of remarkable delicacy and panache — I watched the joy spread from one person to the next in the control room. I felt it myself. Susan and I watched until the James Webb was well on its way, free of the atmosphere, its glorious trajectory precisely on the pre-calculated track. With all that could go wrong in the project, and all that had gone wrong in our society over the past years, here was an elegant response, a human response, that reminded us all of our questing nature and the beauty of science. Unexpectedly, it had been the most memorable Christmas I had experienced in decades.

Meanwhile on earth it had been seven months since my first appointment to check on my shortness of breath; roughly five since I began the Tagrisso regimen. I felt good. Family and friends who telephoned during the holidays mentioned that my voice sounded like my voice from before all of this happened. My weight topped out at about 195, a little plump, honestly, but I discovered, to my amusement, that I was not immune to the societal push for resolutions that the New Year inevitably brings. Vanity apparently can survive cancer! I considered a diet, or at least eating better, and I vowed to exercise more. At the same time, I could not hide from my own eyes the fact that my legs had grown thinner, that my arms and shoulders belonged to an old man. When I went out to shovel snow, or clean off the car, I became winded in no time. I began to think of Tagrisso as a friend, but a supercilious one, a flatterer who could hide the truth from the reality of the situation. Again, I wondered if I was not kidding myself that I had years, potentially, not mere months.

My next appointment, complete with a CT scan and a consultation with Dr. Dragnev, was scheduled for early January. Although I anticipated no surprises, I was aware that the CT scan of my chest might reveal a reversal in my condition. If the pleural effusion had returned, if the cancer had begun to grow again, then I faced a rapidly deteriorating condition. Both Susan and I understood that I was unlikely to accept a round of chemo if the cards came up against me. Enough was enough.

A day before the appointment, my left knee began to hurt. In other times, back in my past, I wouldn't have given it a thought. Anyone in my age bracket is accustomed to the aches and pains of aging. But the knee hurt a good deal, and, more troubling, I could not think of anything that had brought it on. Naturally, I imagined blood clots; I also wondered if cancer could travel to something as innocuous as a knee. I became aware that cancer, unfortunately, could turn one into a small child afraid of any sound in the night. Any discord, any unusual ache, could hold one paralyzed in bed, listening for the crunch of a boot on broken glass from the monster conjured out of the beat and fury of a passing weather storm.

A few days before the appointment, Dartmouth-Hitchcock wrote to say that, due to increased Covid concerns, guests were now restricted. Only the most necessary caregivers were allowed to accompany the visiting patient, and we could not in good faith say that Susan met that standard. I told her several times that she should not take the day off, that we could communicate by phone during my meeting with Dr. Dragnev, but she insisted on accompanying me even though she would not be permitted inside the building.

"It's not something you should do alone," she insisted. "If there's bad news, I don't want you handling that all yourself."

"I really doubt there will be bad news."

"I agree, but to be on the safe side . . ."

Love, I've always thought, is showing up. It's saying yes when no is easier.

On the day of the appointment, she dropped me off at the main entrance to Dartmouth-Hitchcock, then drove off to a nearby grocery/café where she could sit in relative isolation — again, because of Covid — and work until my meeting with Dr. Dragnev.

By this time, my routine at Dartmouth-Hitchcock was established: Blood draw first thing so the results could be uploaded into my portal, CT chest scan in a room across the campus, consultation with Dr. Dragnev, then finish the day with an infusion of the bone-strengthening drug Xgeva, to counteract the calcium-leaching side effect brought on by Tagrisso. Without Susan to keep me company I knew I would have time to kill on my own, so I spent some minutes selecting my reading material and finally settled on Robertson Davies's *Fifth Business*.

*Fifth Business* is the opening volume of the Deptford Trilogy, one of my favorite reads from a lifetime of reading. It follows the life and times of Dunstan Ramsay, a teacher and hagiographer, whose life, from his early days in a Canadian village, is intertwined with those of an illusionist and a sugar beet magnate. It is a masterwork, one I first read in the mid-1980s when I was a teacher in Vienna's American International School. A friend had recommended it, and I had been pulled into it so deeply that it influenced a novella I wrote and which I subsequently published in a story collection titled *A Cup of Stars*. The story was called "The Boar Hunter," set in Vienna and the rural countryside of Austria, and in it I attempted to capture some of the magic and mysticism of Davies's creation.

In any case, going through my day at Dartmouth-Hitchcock, being pinched and prodded with medical tests and soundings, I found I carried the novel in my head. The story starts off with an accident, a hand of fate, when a snowball meant for Dunstan, or Dunny, slams into the head of a pregnant woman and thereby begins a series of events and tragedies that commence with the premature birth of a small son. It is such an economical beginning, so wise and elegant, that I admired it again — forty-plus years after first reading it — as a model of storytelling. It brought Canadian frost into the waiting room and carried me off to a land I didn't know but could imagine. For a time, in between a blood-drawing and the injection of a dye to make the condition of my lung more apparent, I lived in pre–World War I Canada, a simpler time, we're told, but one that is remarkably complex in reality. All of the things I love and loved about reading were folded into the marvelous opening: intelligence, clear writing, splendid character development, a keen eye for observation, and vivid atmosphere. I had always told my students that a novel or story requires a tiger; something real or imagined must be chasing the characters, and Davies's people, I recalled, were chased by destiny and the collision of lives inadvertently giving shape to the lives around them.

It was a compelling juxtaposition. Sitting in a modern facility, surrounded by high-tech machinery, being attended to by nurses and doctors going about their routines, I was able, courtesy of *Fifth Business*, to leave that world and enter another. It was a trade I gladly made. I realized while sitting in the waiting room for Dr. Dragnev's consultation that I had used books all my life for similar quiet escapes. In Africa, during my years in the Peace Corps, my reading habit had deepened and become more important in my life. Stripped of modern conveniences, no TV or consistent radio, and far from the birth of personal computers, we volunteers had traded books as one might trade valuable baseball cards. We knew how important books could be. We read fat books, nineteenth-century novels like *The Count of Monte Cristo*, *The Hunchback of Notre Dame*, *Middlemarch*, and so forth. For Peace Corps volunteers of that era, novels had never been too long or turgid; we lived in the slow, timeless world of West Africa, lived by lantern light and outdoor latrines, airmail letters written on tissue paper, and hotel lobbies with large fans turning overhead.

It was true that Susan could not be with me that day, but I was not alone. I had a book with me and that, as I knew, had always been enough. *Fifth Business* was a portal to the 1900s and the brutality of World War I, but it was also an artifact from the land of the Hardy Boys and *Call of the Wild*, from *Charlotte's Web* and *The Witch of Blackbird Pond*, a close cousin to the countless books whose pages had left their tastes on my fingers. My body might be ill, I granted, but the paper worlds I had visited in my life remained vast and memorable. No matter what happened to me, no matter how the months ahead could shear me, a thousand books waited to rescue me, the simple flying carpet of black print on white pages a friend as trusted as any I had ever encountered.

# 9

Dr. Dragnev asked me how I felt, then listened attentively while I answered. It was a diagnostic tool, I realized, but a necessary one. A patient can be his or her own best diagnostician. I told him I felt fine; that I had a cough sometimes, a loose, phlegmy cough; that my knee had been hurting a few days before; that I grew winded fairly easily; that my appetite was good; that I had indeed put on weight; that my skin had been clear; that I slept well, but sometimes too much; that I felt weaker in everyday tasks; that sleeping on my side, my right side, caused a liquid blockade in my breathing that sometimes would not clear; that my bowels were good; that occasionally I had difficulty retrieving a necessary word or phrase, but that I wasn't sure if that was the product of the cancer, the heavy drugs I took, or simple old age.

"The Tagrisso would not do that," he said after listening. "The brain, I mean. We could do a brain scan to check things. It's possible you've had a small stroke."

"I think I'd rather go forward."

"Then I'll depend on Susan to monitor your word retrieval. Do you hear that, Susan?"

"Yes, I heard that," she said from her post by the phone.

"It takes me a little longer to do a crossword," I added. "And I used to be a pretty good *Jeopardy!* player, but now even if I know an answer, I have difficulty calling it up."

"Let's keep an eye on it."

The good news, however, was that Dr. Dragnev set my next appointment two months into the future. That meant, as we both knew, that I was doing as well as someone in my condition could hope for. Anything could change, of course, and the cancer was far from defeated, but two months — into late February or even early March — made me feel like a schoolboy on the eve of summer vacation.

When Susan picked me up at the front entrance of the hospital, she handed me two cookies she had selected for me. A sugar cookie and a peanut butter cookie. I ate the peanut butter cookie immediately — it was softer than the sugar cookie and a better bet all the way around — and we laughed and told each other we had a place to stand in this cancer journey. As careful as we often were not to jump too far ahead, it was hard not to see hope in the visit with Dr. Dragnev. If he said I was okay, then I was okay. I trusted him, and I trusted my renewed appetite and the pleasure I took in looking out the window at the New Hampshire countryside, covered with snow now. The deep blue-white light of winter surrounded us. In a month, I knew, songbirds would begin to return to scout for nests. With them would come the greater light, the reddening of branches, and the rivers would slowly begin to emerge from their sleeves of ice.

Three days later, while writing the date on a check I was sending out, I realized January 7 marked the fiftieth anniversary of my mother's death. The day itself did not surprise me; I knew that she had died after my first semester in college. I had been home on winter break, and she had slowly succumbed, drifting away into a coma. But fifty years! I knew that it had taken place a long time ago, but the roundness of the fifty figure, the mental framework that quickly translated it as a half century, seemed unfathomable. We often see our own deaths in the death of our parents, but the truth was I had been too young to understand fully what her passing had meant. Now, with my own diagnosis, the anniversary of her death seemed more poignant. I wondered what she had thought and felt about her mortality. She had just entered into the lovely age of grandparenting, a time that, if one is lucky, can be a season of harvest. I could remember her delight as some of my first nephews and nieces arrived at our house for visits, the cribs and scattered diaper bags of my visiting older siblings bringing a fresh, unbridled energy to our home. I remember her rocking the tiny children — how perfect they seemed and how marvelously new! — and leaning forward in her chair to hold their hands while they experimented with walking. Surely, she had not anticipated her early death. Surely, she had hoped to be a grandmother a dozen, maybe two dozen times over. And then in a single summer her diagnosis had arrived and she was gone by January. I hoped, thinking of her on the remembrance of that day, that she had been fully conscious of the hand fate had given her. I hoped that she had looked around her and felt a sense of accomplishment at least as deep as the love that surrounded her. I hoped on her last breath she had felt peaceful and calm, content to turn out the lights and accept what had arrived at last, the end of her, the acceptance of nothingness.

With the turn of the New Year behind us, I began to plan in earnest for our trip to see the sandhill cranes. I had taught beside a colleague who had been raised in Nebraska, and when I had mentioned to her the desire to see the migration, she had shrugged, gave a wry smile, and said something like: *It's a good place to go if you really, really like birds.*

She was not enthusiastic. That time of year in Nebraska — mid-March or early April — can be brutally cold. Furthermore, the cranes are unpredictable. They might arrive earlier or later in the numbers needed to make the migration visually dramatic, depending on weather conditions, and the trip out from New Hampshire would take most of a week. Then, naturally, there was the whole business of hotels, bird blinds (you had to book a reservation to get the best viewing spots), and where to stop along the way. After getting some possible dates from Susan, I began to search through the possibilities, aware that I might be putting more emphasis on the trip than it could support. My colleague had been correct: March in Nebraska did not constitute many people's idea of a vacation destination! I was sensitive, too, to the idea of burning up Susan's vacation days on something as spartan as the trip promised to be. Getting out of late winter in New Hampshire only to travel to a potentially colder location seemed a perverse idea of a getaway.

But Susan and I had a history of enjoying travel that was sometimes adventurous. We had done a camping trip to Yellowstone and points west, and then we had road-tripped it back to the East Coast. The highlight of our travel together had been a four-day raft trip down the Colorado through the Grand Canyon. That trip had struck all of our favorite notes. It had taken a defined time, it had been a chance to "do" rather than simply "see," and it had put us out under the stars in some of the most beautiful landscapes one could find on earth. Susan had said several times after the trip that it was one of the best breaks from everyday life she had ever experienced. I wanted to give her a similar experience with the sandhill cranes. Call it chasing awe. I held a suspicion that a half million cranes, landing, courting, hooting, and clicking their beaks, would make for a memorable event.

Covid, however, worried us. We both understood that if I were exposed to Covid, if I became infected, it might be the end of me. Dr. Dragnev had given us a talk about the potential lethality of the virus, but he had also made the case that we could not be scared and live a satisfactory life. My son put it in a lighter way. He said I could go reclusive Howard Hughes, grow my nails into curled sheaths of keratin, never visit a barber, and mumble my way through bowls of oatmeal, but that was the only way I could guarantee full protection from Covid.

It was a pickle. My last semester in the classroom had been marred by Covid, by the difficulty the students and I had navigating what had then been a new circumstance. We had all adapted by meeting online, but I couldn't persuade myself that it amounted to the same level of teaching and student interaction I had known for three decades. By March, I hoped, the Omicron surge would have begun to subside, but it was impossible to know. Beyond my personal horizon, the world had been going through its own sickness, one that did not seem ready to relent perhaps in my lifetime.

Winter, meanwhile, settled in with a firmness that surprised me. The past few years had been comparatively mild in New Hampshire, but this January the temperature dropped and locked us inside. While I enjoyed what I thought of as an old-fashioned New England winter, the cold air played havoc with my breathing. I used trips to my woodshed as a workout — two loads of cordwood in a plastic sled daily, then transferring it into a wheeled carrier that I tugged inside — and I was able, thereby, to monitor my condition. I grew aware as the days grew marginally longer that I ran out of breath faster during any kind of task. On one particularly cold day, I remember standing and wheezing over the sled, my hands on my hips, the frigid air drawing a bagpipe drone out of my lungs. I watched the birds on my feeder. For some reason we have always had an abundance of cardinals, and I tried to control my breathing as a female pecked at the ground below the feeder, its color — yellowish red, with a corvid crown, a beak the tint of sand — highlighting it against the snowy backdrop. A calendar picture, I supposed. But my breathing did not ease for a long time. It struck me that this type of chore, this New Hampshire existence, would soon be surrendered to cancer. It was not negotiable; there would be no squaring of one's shoulders and facing the difficulties head-on. No stiff upper lip or determined perseverance. Humility was now the order of the day. I would keep bringing in wood and filling the stove on the coldest nights, but I couldn't kid myself that this was sustainable. I would need my son to move in with me permanently, or ask Susan to come and stay. My independence, in other words, was a burning wick. It was not an easy thing to know about myself.

Around this time, I began going to bed with a water bottle. Cold found me more easily than it had in the past, and Susan recommended a red, rubber water bottle as a solution. I laughed at her when she gave it to me, but during this cold January, I fell into the habit of boiling a kettle and pouring the water into the ridiculous bladder. A hot-water bottle! It was the stuff of cartoons and episodes of *The Three Stooges*! But, oh, it was luxury! At bedtime I put the bottle under the blankets while I washed my face and brushed my teeth. By the time I slid into bed the covers had borrowed some of the heat from the bottle and the entire cocoon of blankets was delicious. It was such a simple thing, but it made reading at night — often at two in the morning, when I woke with the wind or to the sound of snow sliding off the roof — a highlight in my day. To be safe in bed, to be warm, to have a good light and a good book, were pleasures that sharpened with the territory I lost to cancer. I read and finished *Fifth Business*, went on to a Pat Conroy memoir about playing point guard for the Citadel, read *Clemmie* by John D. MacDonald and almost anything else that came to hand. Sometimes I coughed and felt the presence of the cancer waiting inside me, but just as often I was able to submerge into the book at hand, the night a promise of dark peace.

I also began reading survival or near-death narratives that I thought, perhaps, might lead me to know what others thought at the moment of their deaths. I was not scientific about my search. I Googled this and that, read what I liked, discarded most entries. For a week or two I became stuck on shipwreck narratives — a genuine phenomenon of the eighteenth century — that made up an entire genre for the seagoing nations of Europe, Britain and Portugal chief among them. Shipwrecks were an everyday experience in that era, and there was no scarcity of hair-raising accounts. The most famous of these narratives was, of course, *Robinson Crusoe*, written by Daniel Defoe and based on the castaway Alexander Selkirk, a Scotsman who survived four years on a Pacific island called Más a Tierra. The shipwreck narratives, the academic critics of such stories pointed out, sought to illuminate national characters, gender considerations, and, frequently, disdain for native peoples. I found them fascinating, but of little value to my circumstances. I searched, I realized later, for stories of people who had begun to die, were saved by a stroke of luck — in my case, Tagrisso — and then went on to live some little while beyond what had appeared to be a predictable death. I rolled the phrase *borrowed time* around in my mind, wondering, under close scrutiny, what the saying actually meant. Wasn't all time borrowed? Or perhaps none of it?

Some of the best contemplations about death came from Michel de Montaigne, the famous French essayist. A skeptic of the first order, Montaigne was not sentimental about death. He provided a simple, straightforward lens with which to regard a life cut short, although he would have mocked the notion of a life being cut or prolonged in any significant way.

> And therefore to lament that we shall not be alive a hundred years hence, is the same folly as to be sorry we were not alive a hundred years ago. . . . Long life, and short, are by death made all one; for there is no long, nor short, to things that are no more.

He also said:

> Life in itself is neither good nor evil; it is the scene of good or evil as you make it. And, if you have lived a day, you have seen all: one day is equal and like to all other days. There is no other light, no other shade; this very sun, this moon, these very stars, this very order and disposition of things, is the same your ancestors enjoyed, and that shall also entertain your posterity.

It was possible, I concluded, to gain some insight by reading these sorts of passages, but I was not sure I trusted them. They were too neat; in their precise language and careful wording they dulled, or diluted, an intensely personal experience. While I did not dread death, neither did I look forward to the final acceptance of its arrival. The few times I had brushed close to death, especially in a near-drowning death off the New Jersey coast, my surrender had not been thoughtful or placid. I did not "die in the mind" as some writers liked to phrase it. No, I had been aware of the water closing over me, of my own weakened body, of the inevitability of the outcome. I had given up, or surrendered, and I could recall, during certain quiet moments in my later life, that it had been a peaceful feeling, but numbing as well. The waves brought me up onto the beach without any power of my own. They had cast me up, a suburban Robinson Crusoe, tossed onto the sand of Point Pleasant, New Jersey, my swim trunks half down on my thighs, my bony fourteen-year-old chest grated and bleeding from a jetty rope to which I had tried to cling in the forceful surf. When I looked up, I did not see anything sacred or romantic. Instead, a small ring of my friends had formed, and they laughed uproariously to see my naked ass and my inelegant tumble onto the beach. Fourteen-year-old boys are merciless creatures, but more to the point, they had not gone through the blue-green ocean water, heard the waves sucking the sand beneath me, felt the liquid gilt of salt and water deep in my lungs. In that way, they were not dissimilar to Montaigne or even to my beloved Marcus Aurelius. We cannot die for anyone else; nor, in the end, can we keep them company or learn from them what is needed. We are all castaways in the final analysis, all survivors who look out to sea and spy no boats arriving, nothing for which to light a signal fire.

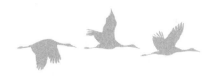

## 10

In earlier winters, I had made a habit of strapping a pair of spiked creepers onto my boots to hike down an abandoned railroad bed at least a half hour a day. It had been a genuine pleasure when I had dogs to walk, but even afterward I still enjoyed the exercise. New Hampshire's winters will eat you if you are not careful to stay active, and part of fighting the seasonal dip of energy and spirits requires we get outside, regardless of the temperature or precipitation. The saying goes that the best way to get warm in New England during the winter is to go outside, because when you return indoors the house feels lovely and warm.

With cancer, however, I was more or less housebound. Despite Melissa Storm's encouragement to walk and get my lungs pumping, I found the attempts to take an afternoon constitutional left me feeling psychologically bruised. To go half a block, stop, breathe with difficulty, then continue, stop, breathe again, reminded me that this condition would not release me. Throughout my life, and especially when I was an active athlete, I had slowly worked my way out of a dozen orthopedic injuries. Ripped tendons across the top of my foot; surgery on my lateral meniscus; helmet blow to the deep blood vessels and meaty tissue of my right thigh; strained vertebrae in my lower back — all injuries from which I had recovered in due course. Mentally, I had never given the injuries a place to stand in my personal universe. Of course I was going to mend; of course I was going to improve. The insult to my body, and to my future level of activity, was temporary and well within my control to address it.

But that was no longer the case. There was no "therapy" for my condition except gently to exhort me to keep moving and remain active. Going to bed or lounging on a couch, as I sometimes gave in to, was seen as self-sabotage. No one would call me out on it — a dubious benefit of such a dire diagnosis, I suppose — but I saw the worry in their eyes. Susan would sometimes ask if I napped, if I had slept late, and so on. Given Covid, given winter, given the fact that if I fell while on the prescribed blood thinners I could readily bruise and bleed in new, concerning ways, I did not lower the drawbridge. I stayed in the castle, eating poorly, indulging in ridiculous television programs — on weekends I distracted myself by watching football games that consumed entire afternoons — and becoming undeniably fussy. My patience was not always what it should be and my interests, and concentration, moved like a wind inside me.

During one of these slack days, I ventured onto my Dartmouth-Hitchcock portal and browsed through my case history. I tended to rely on Susan to relay whatever she thought I should know; she was wonderful at winnowing through the dense medical information and — apart from its effect on our lives — she seemed actually to take an interest in the entire business of tests and results and diagnoses. For my part, I balanced on a fence somewhere between wanting to know everything to the last molecule or wondering if it would prove dangerous to know too much. Willful ignorance, I suppose. Nevertheless, I valued Dartmouth's policy of transparency that gave me access to everything about my case.

I read a little about my recent CT scan to begin. The radiologist gave this report:

Extensive mixed patchy and groundglass left lung paren-chymal opacities generally similar to prior. The differential consideration remains the same, with findings most likely reflecting a combination of inflammatory/infectious and malignant disease.

As before, diffuse, innumerable skeletal metastases.

Hydropic gallbladder.

And this was Dr. Dragnev's visit summary:

I personally reviewed a chest CT showing stable small bilateral pulmonary nodules, no pleural effusion, stable small liver lesions, stable sclerotic changes in the bone lesions, and persistent to slightly more solid ground-glass opacities in the left lower lobe.

Pleural fluid showed adenocarcinoma, PD-L1 1%, not enough material for molecular analyses.

Liquid biopsy — EGFR exon 19 deletion.

### ASSESSMENT AND PLAN:

A 68 y.o. male patient with non-small-cell lung cancer, stage IV, with EGFR activating mutation, receiving osim-ertinib. There was a complete CNS response. There is no progression on today's chest imaging. The left lung opaci-ties are overall stable. This correlates with the clinical improvement, consistent with recovery from an infection, with evolving fibrosis. The appearance is not typical for osimertinib toxicities or malignancy, we will monitor. The treatment is tolerated well. I counseled the patient and his companion (by phone) about the results, their implications for the prognosis as well as the available treatment options. The patient understands that this is an incurable malignancy where systemic treatment is the mainstay. Radiation may be given to palliate symptoms. The goals are survival prolongation as well as quality of life improvement. A balance between side effects and benefits from treatment must be kept. We talked about the benefits of osimertinib, and its side effects were outlined including, but not limited to, skin rash, diarrhea, and the less-common but serious damage to the kidneys, heart, lungs and liver among others. Best-supportive care with emphasis on symptom relief was outlined as an alternative. At this point the patient prefers to continue treatment. Will administer denosumab for bone metastases today, I counseled the patient about the potential toxicities of this agent and the need to take calcium and vitamin D. We discussed the episodes of word-finding difficulties, the potential causes. We reviewed the option of brain imaging now or at the next visit. He prefers the latter unless the symptoms change. I counseled on the risks and benefits of either approach and advised him to call if symptoms change. I counseled on covid-19 precautions. He will come back in 2 months for evaluation. The patient and his partner had numerous questions that were answered to their satisfaction. They agreed with this plan. I advised the patient to call if he develops any fever, shortness of breath, new pain, weakness, bleeding or any other unusual medical symptoms.

What to make of all that?

I read it twice, then turned off the computer and went to fix a cup of tea. As I boiled water, slipped a tea bag in a favorite cup, I wondered at the impersonal nature of the descriptions. I was not referred to by my name; I was a *68 y.o. male patient* with a cancerous condition. As a former English teacher, I took notice of the passive voice. It was impossible to read the notes without understanding that, to a large degree, I was simply one of many patients to pass under the eyes of my cancer team. It made me wonder how Dr. Dragnev, and others in the field, prepared for an appointment. Did they snatch five minutes to refresh themselves about the particulars of my case before we met? While I was meeting Dr. Dragnev or Dr. Backer as a singular person in my life, a meeting under dire circumstances, I was one of many patients they would treat and counsel over the years. I supposed, honestly, that I had experienced a similar relationship with many of my students, though, naturally, the stakes were far more modest. While I certainly tried to be as caring and attentive as I could be with each student, the fact is that they inevitably ran together in my mind. I realized that I had counted on the medical team's personal interest in me rather than as one patient in a parade of patients. Ultimately, my background made little difference. It was not necessary to consider my past, my life's work, my kinship lines in order to treat me. I was patient X with Y symptoms. In their defense, they had demonstrated nothing but warm, kind regard for me and Susan and Justin, but I had missed, or deliberately ignored, the fact that I was the slightly drunken customer talking to a bartender. My concerns and troubles were vividly real to me, but when it came time to describe what they observed in my condition, they reverted to clinical language. They were bartenders wiping the bar with one hand while nodding at yet another story of woe.

Even as I thought these things, I understood I was being horribly unfair. These were just notes I had read, after all. Most likely, the notes served to keep a running record of treatments and findings, while also giving the medical team space to react to what it encountered. The notes also kept my case open for study by others who needed information about me; when I had gone to Portsmouth Hospital to see about my blood clot, the doctors there had been able to speak the same language about my illness. And, finally, the notes probably provided some cover in case of legal questions surrounding a patient's treatment and eventual resolution.

"Do you regret reading them?" Susan asked me when I told her I had spent some time browsing my record.

"No, I don't think so. I'm just not sure how much they help."

"I looked up most of the terms."

"Any new insights?"

"No, pretty much what we already knew."

The language of the reports reminded me of a chemistry set I had been given one Christmas when I was nine or ten. I was not much of an amateur chemist, but the kit came with sufficient equipment, and instructions on how to turn a Ping-Pong table-top into a working lab, so that I had found it an entrance to a little, enticing world. I don't remember doing any experiments — unless waving sulfur powder under friends' noses to show them how bad it smelled counts as an experiment — but I remember sitting at the table, test tubes and glass droppers arrayed around me, and feeling the excitement of a contained focus of study. The kit came with a guide to writing up lab reports, and I remember delighting in the formal template, complete with a space for hypothesis, method, results, and findings, on a tongue of paper that might have served just as well as a detective pad for a game of Clue. I recalled the disembodied voice urged by the chemistry set, the dry, unpopulated prose that set out to make the reports scientific. My patient notes, I realized eventually, represented a grown-up lab report, one that leached all emotion out of the communication and delivered the facts in unadorned transcription valued for its plain, unfiltered renderings. I decided not to read any more case notes unless it seemed absolutely necessary to do so.

Besides, I had other fish to fry. Shortly before the new year, I had applied to AstraZeneca, the manufacturer of Tagrisso, to see if I might qualify for a discount program. I was sixty-eight now, retired, on a fixed income, and the initial payment for the drug, with Medicare, had been $3,000 for the first month and $750 thereafter. I was fortunate that I was able to pay it. The actual cost of the drug, from what I read, was somewhere in the ballpark of $16,000 for a thirty-pill regimen. It was difficult to know what that meant and how it was determined, but when I went online and looked around I found it cost £5,770 in Britain and $8,000 per twenty-eight day course in Canada. Although I was not an experienced drug shopper, I was fairly certain there was no underground Tagrisso market. At least none existed that I could find. As a result, it was either qualify for the discount program or get ready to pay a little more than $11,000 per annum to remain alive.

The application process was complicated, and I wondered, as I had many times, how a patient who was more symptomatic than I would have been able to handle such involved matters. But I pushed through and sent it off, unsure of how I would be notified of the results. Despite the cumbersome application process, I felt enormously grateful to AstraZeneca. It was not an overstatement to say the company — the researchers and technicians, investors and executives — had saved my life. That was not an exaggeration. We often say something like, *Gosh, that was a lifesaver*, or, *Boy, am I glad to see you, you saved my life*, but in this instance it could not have been truer. It struck me as odd that I couldn't thank anyone specifically. The company headquarters, from what I could glean, were in Cambridge, United Kingdom. AstraZeneca describes itself as a global pharmaceutical company, one that was the product of a merger between Swedish company Astra AB and the English company Zeneca Group in 1998.

According to the company publicity literature, "the name Zeneca was invented by a branding consultancy who had been instructed to find a name which was memorable, had no associations with other companies, nor was offensive in any language."

The application submitted, my next medical appointment nearly two months in the distance, that's where things stood for a time. Gradually I realized that now, these days, constituted the "extra time" Tagrisso had bought me. For people who had a specific goal for their waiting — the birth of a grandchild, a trip back to Ireland to trace one's ancestry, a week in Mardi Gras saloons to listen to good jazz — they could point to this interval and connect the temporary victory won by the Tagrisso as the identifiable reason to be grateful. I imagined that even those people, however, used those life events as shorthand to justify the gain of hours and minutes, sunsets and sunrises. From my point of view, this quiet time of deep January reminded me of the several times I had jumped off a cliff into water below. Once, in Negril, Jamaica, I had climbed to the top of a rocky outcropping then climbed again into a tree that hung out over the water. After establishing my balance, and checking the water below, I leaped perhaps fifty feet into the pure blue of the Caribbean. What I recalled was the initial excitement of leaving the earth, then, just as quickly, the momentary peace of falling, the air sliced on either side of me, my body relaxed but ready, the horizon falling with me as I approached the earth. To strain the metaphor, I had climbed the height of cancer, balanced myself, then jumped. The water waited, but for now, for this little time, I was suspended, neither of earth nor air, a boy falling with his hands crossed against his chest.

One evening while watching *Jeopardy!*, I happened to channel-hop during a commercial to a local show called *New Hampshire*

*Chronicle.* The show follows two attractive young hosts, a male and a female, as they sample the pleasures and oddities of the Granite State. They might trap a nuisance bear one week with the local Fish & Game, go on a dogsled loop around the Mount Washington hotel the next, or simply visit a chocolatier who has opened a new store in an unusual location. Between segments Fritz Wetherbee, an avuncular old-timer in a bow tie, provides brief history lessons concerning a court case adjudicated here, an avalanche there, a log drive on such and such a river. The entire program lasts a half hour and is as easy to swallow as a marshmallow.

On this particular night I was about to switch back to *Jeopardy!* when a segment came on concerning *green burials*. I had heard the term before, but I had never paid much attention. To my surprise and delight, I knew the woman being interviewed about green burials, and, more remarkable, I knew the man who had been buried and who formed the subject of the story. His name was Chris Buckley and he was a wonderful, wonderful man. I knew he had died; I had exchanged emails with him not long before his own lung cancer had taken him. He was a teacher, a writer, an arborist, an outdoorsman, a reader, and a local advocate for environmental living. He was also a husband and partner, a father to a pair of boys who thought the world of him. For one brief semester, I had worked with him on his manuscript, the story of an incredible trip he and his brother, Brandon, took to Labrador when they were naive youngsters filled with wanderlust. It was a grand, rollicking tale, but Chris struggled to find the way to tell it. He modeled his effort on *Great Heart*, his favorite adventure book, written by two New England canoeists, John Rugge and James W. Davidson, which traced the story of three Labrador excursions, and their overlapping crews, in the early 1900s. Chris had recommended the book to me many years back, and it had also become a favorite of mine. A signed copy of the book — which I found in a thrift store — is one of my most valued literary treasures.

In any event, this was Chris, my friend and onetime student, who was somewhere under the soil while the show interviewed Jen, his widow, about home burials. As I followed the program about Chris and green burial, I discovered that Jen had him buried in his backyard, a practice I had heard about but hadn't actually envisioned. There were rules: no cement vault, no embalming, no casket or burial vessel that was not biodegradable. The idea of working with nature, and perhaps being placed in my own land, appealed to me. We had buried many dogs and cats in the backyard, simply wrapping them in an old sheet and putting them well into the ground. It seemed the simplest method with which to dispose of a body, to dispose of me, and in my life I had often found that simplicity meant beauty and grace.

To be earth or air?

That seemed to be part of the question. Ultimately, I doubted it mattered. The moment death arrived, consciousness departed. Beyond that final moment, the body became nothing more than materials returning to the universe. That said, however, I did not like the notion of decomposition, of earth covering my mortal remains. Frankly, I would have preferred what is sometimes called an open burial, or a sky burial as it's known in the Himalayas. Lay me out on a piece of wilderness and walk away. Let animals make use of what is left behind; let the body be consumed directly, scattered by hunger.

In a little touch of irony, the land we had purchased in Maine contained the body of a woman who had died — stories differ about its origin — aboard a ship up from Boston or maybe Nova Scotia. Her name was Harriet Carr, and the grave waited in the middle of the property, alone and unaffiliated with any cemetery or church. Shortly after I took possession of the land, I called the Pembroke Historical Society and asked if they knew anything about the grave. They were perplexed to hear of it, and two members, a married couple, came out to look at it. We spent an hour on our hands and knees, propping up the headstone that had cracked and fallen backward, weeding, and wetting paper towels to drag across the inscription in order to read it more clearly. We pieced together what we could, and later, the woman of the couple emailed me to say she had done some research and felt pretty confident that Harriet Carr's husband had moved to Lubec after the death of his wife. He remarried. It was also possible, she said, that Harriet Carr had died in childbirth, and that, possibly, the child had been buried with her.

After I got the news, I wondered whether it was my duty to restore the grave site. I didn't know it existed when I bought the property. Or, from a larger perspective, to clear the grave site of all the granite markers to allow Harriet Carr to release her elements to the universe in peace and obscurity. She had been dead since sometime in the 1840s, and whatever she had been, what memory anyone held of her, had evaporated long ago. In fact, I realized if I removed her stone and let the grave turn back to meadow, she would be gone, once and for all, from all recollections on earth. It was possible there were legal questions surrounding the treatment of a grave, but I understood that by removing the stone and letting the lupines grow thick around her, I could bring about her complete oblivion.

# 11

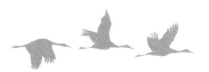

My first memory of life occurred when I was a small child, under age five, on a brick breezeway in Baltimore, Maryland. The breezeway connected the house to the garage. The cement walkway was covered by a roof, but the walls were low, purposefully so to allow air to move through the sultry Baltimore summers. I suppose my mother let me play out there, well within her supervisory radius, where she could peer out the screened door to check on me to make sure I hadn't wandered. Perhaps, as I think of it, she propped something in front of the entrance and exit, turning it into a large, comfortable playpen. In any case, my first memory revolves around stepping outside and becoming aware, for the first time, of my independence. It may be a fantasy, but I recall holding the door open with my left hand while reaching my foot down to the walkway surface. Then, just to the left and carefully framed by the square of the screened door, I saw several large black beetles clustered in the corner of the breezeway.

End of vision. I have no more memory than that. It was fragmentary at best, and who knows whether it is remotely accurate? I have confirmed with my brothers and sisters that there was indeed a brick breezeway, and also that it was the common access we used to come and go. Turn left and you entered the garage; turn right, the house. When I asked if beetles were often found on the porch, they collectively shrugged. It was not something they remembered, and it suggested to me, in my darker moments, of something strange and Freudian about my first memory. After all, why would one recall so vividly the shape and the vibrancy of the black beetles as they clustered in the corner of the breezeway? Surely such a first memory, if it was in fact a true first memory, suggested a burdened mind. The amateur psychologist in all of us can tear the memory apart. Why the ambivalence of standing in the doorway, half out, half in, the screen ready to release me or pull me back inside? And why was this a vision of independence? And what in the world did the beetles represent, if they represented anything, and what kind of beetles had they been?

All of this is to say that the idea of memory, of what we can recall with accuracy, and what is merely a way to color inside the lines of a rough sketch of our life, occupied me frequently in the time after my diagnosis. For many years I have been haunted — although *taunted* might be a better word — by an experience I had while working at the old Stanley Hotel in Estes Park, Colorado. I was somewhere around twenty at the time. I had landed there while hitchhiking around the country and I had secured a job as an all-around go-for. The hotel provided a dormitory for staff on the back grounds of the property, and it was an attractive place for a summer stay. This was the time of John Denver's Colorado anthems, and to be in the mountains, in the lovely old hotel, was payment enough for most young people.

I was an elevator operator, a towel-boy, a bringer of replacements for burned-out lightbulbs. I stayed busy and only learned later that the Stanley Hotel was the setting for Stephen King's *The Shining*. It made sense. The long, dim hallways, and the formidable ballroom and lobby, invited stories of ghosts and isolation. Often during my stay at the Stanley, I felt on edge and a bit anxious that I was not alone when no one else was present.

As part of our payment, the staff was fed before the evening dinner service, usually a hodgepodge of leftovers and ersatz lodge dinners. One evening, after being served, someone in our group asked the cook for butter. The cook, a wild-haired, grumpy old man who split his time between Colorado in the summer and Arizona in the winter, told us he was not going to give us butter until whoever put a cigarette out in the butter the night before confessed to doing so.

We were stunned. The room became still as he slid a plate of butter onto our table with the stale cigarette jabbed into the center. I recall that the cigarette had wicked moisture up into its white paper and that the angle of the stab had been almost sideways, as if the perpetrator had stood as he extinguished his cigarette and hurried off. It was obviously a wanton waste of food, and we all looked around, dumbfounded and confused, annoyed that someone had put us in this position.

I glanced around, too. I also felt sharp irritation at whoever had done such a thoughtless thing. I also felt the room tilting to reject the coward who refused to admit what he had done. Then the moment passed, and we resumed our dinner without the benefit of butter.

Ten years, twelve years, a long time afterward, I remembered that I had been the one to stab the cigarette into the butter.

Strange, perhaps. I am fairly certain that the other diners knew I had done it. The brand of cigarette, a Newport menthol, was my brand of smoke. In that instant, however, when I was confronted with my misdeed, I suppressed all memory of my action and looked around the room as innocently as any other member of our party. If someone had held a gun to my head and ordered me to confess, I would have taken the bullet. I had done nothing wrong. The butter was not something I would befoul.

Looking back, the story seems somewhat innocent. It was merely a stick of butter, for goodness' sake, and I've always wondered if the cook saw me do it, or if he had taken a dislike toward me. I could also recall that we had smoked in our college cafeteria (many professors smoked in class and sometimes bummed cigarettes from us), often dousing our cigarettes in glasses of milk or pooled salad dressing. The entire practice had been abhorrent and wasteful, but we had performed it casually with no particular ill intent. It was what we did; it's what every smoker in the cafeteria did. In my final reckoning of the event, I realized I had probably stabbed out the cigarette without conscious purpose, had probably been impatient to be outside again after a long day of work. Maybe it was a way of working out some aggression — we were paid horribly and worked hard — but I imagined it was primarily motivated by laziness and a general sloppiness.

But I had not been able to own the memory when I had been confronted by the cook. What else, I wondered, had I suppressed over the years? And how much of what I remembered was accurate?

Along these lines, after hearing of my diagnosis a number of people asked me if I wanted to contact people from my past. For instance, I had not spoken to my divorced wife, Amy, in the better part of thirty years. Susan wondered if I had an interest in contacting her. Propriety of some stripe suggested I should let her know; we were married once and had meant a great deal to each other at one time. I wondered, however, why the compression of a life, knowing the end approached, fueled a desire to see equations balance out. If I had not felt it necessary to be in contact with Amy for thirty years, why would I seek her out now? Did I imagine a consoling conversation between us, something that would put us both at peace? I mistrusted the impulse.

Besides, where did one stop? Did I contact old girlfriends, my childhood buddy Monte, my good friend from the Peace Corps, Tom, college roommates? It struck me as manipulative. I would knock, metaphorically, on their doors and announce that I had come to say goodbye, that I was dying, that they better decide, once and for all, what they thought about me.

I did not want another opinion about the memorable moments of my life. I allowed myself an inventory of memories — false or not — that seemed to demand recollection. I did not filter the memories into good or bad piles, but merely became somewhat skilled at letting them project onto my consciousness. For example, I remembered my brother Chuck leaping toward a basketball goal and coming down on one of our two beagle puppies, Bess, who let out a pitiable cry and lost her life; a policeman shining his light into the back of an old Buick where I had parked with my high school girlfriend, both of us half dressed; a telegram from my father coming while I was in Mali, West Africa, to let me know a short story I had written had won an award in a national contest; the slap of our fifth-grade teacher's marine swagger stick onto his desk at the front of the room, Mr. Gaggliardi, who called us to attention to announce the president of the United States, John F. Kennedy, had been shot; and the angora sweater worn by Cindy, the first girl I had ever held in my arms, in a potato-chip-filled basement party sometime in ninth grade.

Was that the tally of my life? Those memories and more? Did I lack the courage — as Eliot's Prufrock did — to risk misunderstanding?

> *And would it have been worth it, after all,*
> *Would it have been worth while,*
> *After the sunsets and the dooryards and the sprinkled*
>     *streets,*

*After the novels, after the teacups, after the skirts that trail*
*    along the floor —*
*And this, and so much more? —*
*It is impossible to say just what I mean!*
*But as if a magic lantern threw the nerves in patterns on a*
*    screen:*
*Would it have been worth while*
*If one, settling a pillow or throwing off a shawl,*
*And turning toward the window, should say:*
*    "That is not it at all,*
*    That is not what I meant, at all."*

It's undeniably pretentious to quote Eliot, especially Prufrock, but his question was relevant: Did I dare disturb the universe? I imagined turning to Amy to ask if she remembered this or that, and if she remembered it as I remembered it, only to have her shake her head softly and put forth a different rendition. Would I be seeking confirmation of my version of events, or a different lens through which the moments of my life might get greater clarity? It did not seem a journey worth taking. Something about dying tempted us to lose the core of ourselves. I did not want to end like a man whose paper bag full of groceries ripped on the way to the car, clutching and trying to patch things as I went, covering the unfixable holes with panicked hands. No, whatever I had been, however I had triangulated life to this point, seemed to be the better track to take.

Ted, Bob, and I rented a place near the Vermont border to watch football together in the middle of the month. Although we were casual fans, we selected the NFL's best weekend — two games on Saturday, two on Sunday — with what we hoped were well-matched teams. Bob and I had played football together many years before, and Ted, who had been affiliated as an academic adviser with the University of Connecticut's championship basketball teams, loved sports and the trash talking of athletes. Amid a long, cold New England winter, it was an excuse to get away.

It occurred to me as I drove over to Grantham, New Hampshire, that I was now roughly seven months beyond the first news of cancer. Maybe eight months. The shape of a year with cancer had begun to form in me. It was a phrase people used: *He's two years cancer-free. He's a cancer survivor of five years.* Such phrases met a human need to quantify time, I supposed, to put it in a sturdy basket with handles. Living eight months after my cancer diagnosis, was I now a survivor? When did one transition from being a patient with cancer to being a survivor? It struck me as a fuzzy calculation. Some medical texts called for a certain number of years to have passed in order to be called a survivor; others suggested from the day you received a cancer diagnosis you were a survivor. A designation that lumped in a twenty-year survivor with someone a mere eight months past the first CT scan seemed less than useful.

The flip side of the thought was that, sans Tagrisso, I would have already been dead two or three months. I doubted I would have lived long past Halloween. In a strange sense — and I felt this strongly — I was a ghost of myself. I had been pulled back from death by a pill made by a company I had never heard of, had benefited from a biochemical interaction I could not begin to explain, had been saved by a genetic mutation that was rare among Caucasian men, had escaped the promise-filled poisons of chemotherapy, and had landed here, in a car driving to join two old friends in a silly ritual of football watching. I felt like Scrooge when he wakes from his haunting to find it is still Christmas Day. I was alive; the past was secured away and the future, foreboding as it might be, had not yet found me. Unlike Scrooge, however, I could not call to a passing boy out my window and send a prize turkey to Bob Cratchit. I could not make any firm resolutions about the future, turn over a new leaf, become something other than my own ghost.

We had rented one of those brown-beamed condos that are beloved by Massachusetts skiers who drive up Route 91 and think they have entered heaven if the rental has a fireplace. It was comfortable and warm and had adequate seating for three large men. It took us a half hour, and several YouTube videos, to figure how to turn on the television, but by early evening we were solidly parked in front of the first game, drinking beer and laughing at the ancient, familiar stories that bubbled up whenever we got together. We talked about family and we talked about fishing the following spring, and we welcomed the interruptions the game afforded us, the quick, heroic run by a gifted halfback, or the beautiful spiral cast by a quarterback like a twisting drill bit to a diving receiver. As much as I loved these men, as much as they had been my comrades for a half century, I felt myself drifting away from them. It was not dramatic and it did not merit discussion. Laughing with them, watching the game, fetching beers for one another, it felt like watching a loved one depart across the tarmac to a waiting plane in a different age. You waved and blew a kiss, but a decision of parting had already been made. They climbed the gangway into the fuselage while you watched for a significant sign, an indication that you might be remembered, that this division did not have to be final, although you suspected it was. Then, seeing the hatch close behind them, you waited anyway, watched the plane taxi across the runway, stayed even long enough to watch the plane lift off the ground, as if by watching it you could guarantee its safety, or the impermanence of your separation from one you loved.

# 12

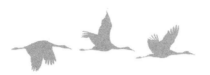

"Most people get a slower runway into this kind of thing. People hear they have a type of cancer and then they have a long series of consultations that say if you do this or that you stand a chance of getting a certain type of outcome. Sometimes it's operable. Sometimes it starts out as Stage One and gradually worsens. Sometimes people are cured if they can simply endure the chemotherapy long enough. But you didn't get anything that was junior varsity. You got the full treatment right from the start."

This is what Susan explained to me after I had fought her about mac & cheese.

If that sounds ridiculous, it's because it was. She had come up for a long weekend to my house in central New Hampshire, and on her way she had stopped at the grocery store to get the fixings for a gourmet batch of mac & cheese. She had a recipe from a well-known chef, and she offered to make me enough so that I could put some in the freezer for a quick meal. Pull one out, nuke it, and voilà. Who wouldn't like a freezer filled with a few mini-vats of mac & cheese?

"I don't need it," I said, rudely.

"Well, I thought it might be —"

I cut her off. I said something like this:

"You worry about me walking on ice and you tell me I should have a railing on the basement steps and I'm okay, Susan. I am.

You can't mother me. I know I have cancer, but I'm okay. The freezer is full and I can eat an egg sandwich just as easily. It's not important to me. I appreciate your help, but I don't need it, honestly."

She regarded me closely. Then she explained, in detail, why I was being a horse's ass.

What I understood was that I apparently needed to push her away. Not far. I needed her too much, counted on her too much, loved her too much to push her very far. Before I had spoken to her and proved myself an idiot, I had no idea I harbored strong feelings about mac & cheese. Of course, the truth was I didn't have any feeling at all about mac & cheese. I knew some Tuesday afternoon in the middle of February I would be glad to reach into the freezer for a quick dinner.

What I rejected was the possibility, the absolute likelihood, that I needed help. That I needed guidance. That the man I had been in my youth and middle years now required someone to fill up his freezer. That someone needed to keep an eye on the level of ice on my driveway, or the rickety nature of the basement steps. I knew my son dropped by often to check on me, to see if he could do anything that would be difficult for me to accomplish, and I knew Susan and he communicated via text about my health. As a former English professor, it reminded me of Regan's statement to her father and liege, King Lear, when she points out that he needs governance.

> **Regan.** *O, sir, you are old!*
> *Nature in you stands on the very verge*
> *Of her confine. You should be rul'd, and led*
> *By some discretion that discerns your state*
> *Better than you yourself.*

Nature in you stands on the very verge of her confine.

It was time for me to be ruled. With increasing frequency, it was possible that Justin and Susan knew more precisely what I needed than I knew myself. It was Justin who warmed a frozen pipe with a hair dryer; it was Susan who carried the laundry basket down the treacherous basement steps in order to save me a trip. While I was grateful for the care and affection behind their actions, I was also aware I had taken my hand off the ship's wheel. If I had ever been a captain — which was doubtful — I was clearly one no longer. To become old is to hand over duties and responsibilities, and that was, embarrassingly and rudely, why I had protested Susan's kind offer to fill my freezer with food.

I apologized a little later. Confessed I was a perfect dope. And we went on.

But I knew King Lear well enough, and I couldn't escape the rough reflection I found in the play. The plot outline goes like this: Lear, who is in his eighties and has tired of his duties as a monarch, decides to divide his kingdom among his three daughters. To gain his good graces, Regan and Goneril plump him up with false flattery and declarations of excessive love, but the good and true Cordelia says she loves him as she is bonded by her filial duty, no more and no less, and that she will save half her love for her future husband. Lear becomes furious at Cordelia's response and divides his kingdom between his two duplicitous daughters, Regan and Goneril, who privately see him as a silly old man. He expects them to feast and revere him, and to maintain his retinue of one hundred knights, but instead finds he is diminished and humiliated and goes slowly mad.

King Lear's hamartia, or tragic flaw, is his arrogance and excessive pride. He lacks self-knowledge, and it is his undoing. Like Lear, I knew I was not immune from the arrogance of the healthy and able. Although I did not have a kingdom to divide, until this last half year I had my health and autonomy as a personal preserve. To give it away, piece by piece, had gradually emptied me until, at last, I misguidedly pushed back against Susan's kind offer to stock my freezer. I made a poor King Lear. Or rather, King Lear and I shared qualities that did not put a good light on either of us.

That was a low point in January. February arrived, and with it, stronger light and longer days. Years ago, I had learned that songbirds returned in February and began searching for nest sites and potential mates before the average homeowner had begun to track them. To scout for them, I went out around noon for several days running and sat in the sun. I waited for the birds while I soaked up the strengthening sunlight and was eventually rewarded by a flock of robins zooming in like college kids returned from spring break in the tropics. It lifted my heart. In prior days, I would have had a book with me, or perhaps my phone, but cancer had given me a peculiar gift — I could now sit in perfect peace and watch the world pass by. The wind still came cold and brisk, but I found a lee side beside a woodshed and sat like the worst parody of an old pensioner on a park bench in any city of the world.

As I sat, I thought about the platitudes that claim cancer, or any deadly disease, can make the world dearer to the struggling patient. In some ways it reminded me of the saying that the fishing is good when it's raining. I've fished enough to know that isn't provably true; it had always struck me as a way to pretend the rainfall is not as unpleasant as it feels. No, from my experience cancer does not bring any particular clarity about life to which I could point. No big, shining lesson, in other words. I was not now able to say what *really counts in life* any more than I had ever been suited to make such a proclamation. I knew a few things that counted for me — watching the robins land and quarrel, feeling the sun on my bones qualified as things that counted for me — but cancer had provided no magical key. I did not sit like the Buddha under the Bodhi tree now experiencing enlightenment. I remained inside my skin, as deeply flawed and as imperfect a human as anyone who had ever been born.

What I did feel, and what is probably inevitable for humans who have discovered the ending to their story must experience, was what is called in German *Torschlusspanik*. It's an intriguing word that means, literally, "gate-shut-panic." In medieval times, if one foolishly failed to get inside the castle before the sun went down and the large drawbridge gate swung home, then one was vulnerable to anything that might happen during the night. Highwaymen, petty thieves, or big bad wolves. It is the fear that the time to act is running out; it's the fear of the ice cream truck's bell disappearing down the block, or the nervous disappointment one might feel as the last present is unwrapped on Christmas morning and the hoped-for gift has still not appeared.

*Torschlusspanik*: I acknowledged its existence. Whatever plans I had promised myself, or Susan, for the future, illness had now made me peer over my shoulder to see the drawbridge ascending. Whatever I wanted to do needed to be done soon or forgotten forever. The drawbridge, heavy and gray-beamed with black iron hardware marking its strength, was slowly swinging up. Like other cancer patients, or patients of any terminal illness, I was destined to spend the night beyond the castle walls, prey to random misfortune, no longer one of the keep's citizens, but rather a stranger whose travel has left him on the wrong side of safety's door.

# 13

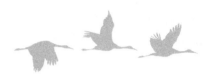

What is death?

The question isn't as silly, or as juvenile, as it sounds. In fact, the idea of death — not merely the cessation of life, but the depiction of death in stories and myth — occupied me a great deal in the early part of February. I wondered if there was something to be gained by reading about death, especially in myth and fairy tale, that might at least allow me to understand its place in our Western culture. The word *death* is so much a part of our language that it had never before occurred to me to wonder anything about it.

*Death comes. We die. He is dead. He was dead when he hit the floor. I die, she exclaims. Death waits for us. Death is around the corner. Dead as a doornail. Death becomes her. Dead reckoning. You will be the death of me. You are dead to me. Only things certain are death and taxes. Drop dead. Drop-dead gorgeous. Little death. Death was a good career move.*

The very word *death* somehow blocks, or obscures, the full import of the physical event. It is a convenient abstraction, a stand-in for the profound physical changes that the cessation of life brings about. We stop short of speaking the truth about death: that it is the beginning of rot, that our profound dissolution begins in the instant of our last breath. John Brown's body may be "a-moldering in his grave," but we don't like to put too fine a point on it. The song continues that his "soul goes marching on," asking us to pretend a soul exists in the first place, and that it goes on in any significant manner in the second. The word *death* is a cultural movie screen, a word that covers the true nature of our demise with whatever projections we decide to shine on it.

In Old English, death is *deaþ*, in Proto-Germanic *dauthuz*, in ancient Saxon *doth*, Old Frisian *dath*, Dutch *dood*, High German *Tod*, Old Norse *dauoi*, Danish and Swedish *Dod*. It's easy to see the transformation of the word into the modern *death*.

As an animate character, death is often depicted either as a dealmaker — he will give something to get something, typically a soul — or as a trickster who can occasionally be bested by clever humans. Usually depicted as male (although not always), the Grim Reaper, a skeletal figure with a long, beckoning finger, is implacable. He cannot be turned away once he sets his sights on someone, although he can be confused or pointedly delayed.

One of the most common tropes in the stories I read is the futility of trying to escape death. We all know this type of story. A person learning that he or she is to die, escapes to a town other than their own and believes she or he is safe. Then, miraculously, the person runs into Death in the new town. When Death is asked how he found the person, Death confesses that he had never searched for the victim in the original town; it is the biting irony of the victim's escape that brought her to Death's final reckoning. Running from death, she ran into Death's arms.

Understandably, much of death's shape and meaning is derived from our culture. In my reading, I was reminded that as a Peace Corps volunteer in West Africa, we learned a fundamental difference between American culture and the culture of Burkina Faso, my host country. In that part of Africa, we were instructed as trainees, all deaths are caused. That seems like a simple statement until you unpack it. People do not die merely from physical causes; the causes themselves are set in place by others, sometimes ancestors, who will the death of the dying person. The result of such a transactional philosophy can be fraught with paranoia and feud. If every time a person dies, we must look to her or his surrounding community to discover the agent of death, it can be an invitation to revenge and mayhem. Witchcraft — charges for and against — is a fact of life in much of West Africa.

In fairy tales and myths, death is often consolidated and made to contend with the protagonist. In the Brothers Grimm story "Godfather Death," a man who has become a father for the thirteenth time despairs that he can feed his children. He runs to the path in front of his hut and offers the newborn — as a godchild — to God, first, then to the Devil. He rejects them both. He rejects God because God gives to the rich and takes from the poor; he rejects the Devil because the Devil leads men astray. At last Death passes by and agrees to stand as godfather for the infant. Not only is Death nonplussed by the offer — he has never been offered anything like it before — but he goes one better and vows to make the boy a famous physician. The boy will be able to cure any illness, no matter how dire, except when he arrives at the deathbed and finds Death waiting at the foot. If Death is at the head of the bed, then the ill person will recover. Death, in other words, must be paid and obeyed.

We anticipate by the tried-and-true arc of the fairy-tale narrative what will happen. The boy will grow into a man and be successful for a time, but then he will transgress and ignore Death's stipulation. And indeed, the godson saves the king from a mortal illness, but in the process disobeys Death by ignoring his presence at the foot of the bed. Death warns the godson in no uncertain terms that the next time he disobeys Death's command it will be the end of him. The king's daughter, whom the physician loves, naturally, becomes ill shortly afterward and the physician again defies Death. Death cannot abide such disobedience and takes the godson in place of the dying princess and shows him a cave where the walls are lined with candles. The candles represent the lives of everyone on earth. Death points to the godson's candle, which is now only a pool of wax, and lets the wick burn out. The godson falls down dead, and Death is respected once more.

It's a curious tale, one that is retold in variant forms through most of Europe. It is a classic depiction of Death, who, in the reading of it, remains rather matter-of-fact. He does not gloat at the godson's death; neither does he show much appetite for destruction. He is a natural force, like wind or fire, and it made me wonder about the effect our stories have on us. In most of the stories I encountered, it is usually the case that — as Kübler-Ross had told us — we look to strike a deal with death. We try to come to acceptable terms. In the back of our minds, however, we know such deals are pocked with treachery. Even if we suspect they will not work, we forge them anyway. We try to cheat Death while Death, in most instances, laughs at our perfidy.

The story that meant the most to me, Hans Christian Andersen's "The Emperor's Nightingale," made the unusual claim that beauty could vanquish death. That suited me. I have always loved the fairy tale, and I can remember reading it and getting teary-eyed as a boy. What I responded to then, I suppose, was the self-sacrifice and nobility of the nightingale. If you recall the story, the emperor of China learns from his court that the sweetest sound in the land is the song of the nightingale. The emperor summons the bird to his castle, but only the kitchen maid knows where to find the bird. The entire court moves to a viewing spot, and the nightingale agrees to sing. The emperor is charmed. Each night the nightingale serenades the emperor, but then the emperor receives a mechanical bird that can sing just as sweetly as the original bird. All works well for a while — I have to say the pond ice is always cracking under the feet of fairy-tale characters — but then, of course, the mechanical bird breaks down. For want of the glad singing, the emperor sinks closer and closer to death, while the people around him look on with futility.

Death, at last, comes and squats on the emperor's chest. This is how it is written in the fairy tale, first published in 1843.

> Opening his eyes he saw it was Death who sat there, wearing the Emperor's crown, handling the Emperor's gold sword, and carrying the Emperor's silk banner. Among the folds of the great velvet curtains there were strangely familiar faces. Some were horrible, others gentle and kind. They were the Emperor's deeds, good and bad, who came back to him now that Death sat on his heart.
>
> "Don't you remember?" they whispered one after the other. "Don't you remember — ?" And they told him of things that made the cold sweat run on his forehead.
>
> "No, I will not remember!" said the Emperor. "Music, music, sound the great drum of China lest I hear what they say!"

But whatever music he summons, it fails to drown out the whispers. Then the authentic nightingale arrives, having heard of the emperor's illness. The bird sings so beautifully that the phantoms around the emperor begin to fade and even Death stops to listen. The nightingale bargains for the emperor's life. Death, at last, departs.

The story is far more nuanced than I realized as a child. Yes, the original nightingale is heroic in the best sense. The bird forgives the emperor's arrogance; it also forgives and quiets the emperor's sins and small voices. I wondered, however, what to make of the emperor himself? Perhaps he was greedy for wishing to possess a form of beauty that was both rare and commonplace to his kingdom. In his defense, perhaps he was a busy man, so having a mechanical contraption makes a certain amount of sense. Of course, he was also faithless. He turned the nightingale's gift away, assuming it could be reproduced with little effort. He was not a true friend to the nightingale. He accepted tribute without volunteering tribute in return. Death, in this instance, acted as a teacher.

It is also a common theme in fairy tales to have Death appear in clothes that mirror the habiliment of the victim. In the nightingale story, Death wears the outward embellishments of an emperor. It is a form of mockery, really, because the sword and crown and silk banner will soon be of little use to the dying emperor. The emperor is not only close to death, but he is also losing his identity.

So, what was my story to account for death? What sort of conflict does he or she afford me as the protagonist of my own life? How did I picture death in my mind, if I pictured it at all?

Although I searched my mind, and even made observational notes to hone my thinking about death, capital *D*, I had difficulty visualizing it. Death was not a person, I decided, nor an entity, but a process instead. I remember learning when I was a preteen about people in comas being buried alive in coffins. The idea terrified and fascinated me. The fear of being buried alive is known as *taphephobia*, and Poe's story "The Premature Burial" revolves around this fear. The narrator, who suffers from catalepsy, worries that he will be mistaken for dead and buried before he can be revived.

I asked a priest about it once, and he confirmed that people did, in fact, wake in their coffins, especially during the cholera epidemic in the Victorian Age; that was the purpose of mortuary bells sometimes erected near a recent burial. If a person regained consciousness soon after being interred, she or he could reach for a dangling cord and make the bell ring. The priest even told me that certain individuals had been stripped of sainthood, because, having come awake in their graves, they did not accept their situation peacefully, trusting in God, but instead dug at the coffin tops and shredded their nails. Upon exhumation, the church assumed that the corpse had despaired in God, and therefore could not be a true saint.

That was the kind of stuff that rattled around in my brain. Again, however, death was not a figure in these musings, but a process. Except for the pleasure fairy tales and myths gave me, death failed to materialize in any meaningful way for me. I was heartened, finally, by a tale of Death appearing to a mortally ill princess, where he arrived as a figure of fear and loathing. But when Death went to visit a desperately impoverished old woman at the edge of her life, he discovered he was an honored guest, one for whom the poor woman had been waiting. She had had enough of life. She went with him willingly, content and at peace. No nightingale sang for her salvation, and Death treated her gently and with respect.

For several days during that same period, I attempted to fill out my calendar for the upcoming spring and summer. I was aware it was premature and somewhat foolhardy given the unpredictability of my illness, but I discovered I needed events to populate what had become a string of empty dates except for doctors' appointments. Besides, these activities had been a large part of my plan for retirement. I told myself that I was alive until I was dead, which is the kind of phony pep talk I usually avoided. If I really bought the idea that I was "alive until I was dead," wouldn't

I begin writing something new, or start doing more sit-ups? Wouldn't I buy a new dishwasher?

In any case, I spent a long time forming travel plans — as I've mentioned — for Susan and me to go to Kearney, Nebraska, in late March to watch the annual migration of sandhill cranes. I booked flights, hotels, rented a car. As kind as Susan is and was, when I reported my bookings I saw in her eyes her concern that I put more into these plans than necessary. She listened patiently to the itinerary, nodded, and told me it all sounded good, but underneath her calm expression I detected her worry. I suppose in my mind I made the bargain that if I could plan to see cranes, I couldn't die. The details of the trip grew in proportion to the emptiness of other demands on my time.

I booked a June camping week at Lake Francis State Park in northern New Hampshire from which I could access some of my favorite fishing spots. With Ted and Bob, we booked a reservation on Maine's Kennebago watershed for spring fishing. I made rough plans to travel to Charleston, South Carolina, in April to see the city and visit one of Susan's daughters. I sketched out an itinerary for a fall fishing safari, complete with stops at Yellowstone's Cave Falls and Sylvan Lake, then Idaho's Kelly Creek and the St. Joe River. I called a builder I knew in Pembroke, Maine, and floated past him several ideas about improving my property there.

The dates and planned activities were a way to declare that I would be healthy enough to experience them. Lacking a secure future, I could line up an outline and hope to fill in the rest of the story later. If Susan was wise to me, and I was sure she was, she didn't say anything. I was a retired guy spending too much time sweeping my porch. Moreover, I was a retired guy with terminal cancer and an unspecified amount of time.

I was in this "make plans" mind-set when the volunteer coordinator of New Hampshire CASA contacted me to see if I was still interested in serving as a guardian ad litem for kids dangling in the state court system. She was kind about checking on me; she was clearing the books for the new year and assessing the future needs of the organization. I was, after all, a certified CASA volunteer who had gone through three months of training, but the diagnosis had arrived at the same moment as my retirement, so the chance to serve on a case never jelled. I had made excuses and promises to myself — after this appointment with Dr. Dragnev, I would get involved, after that test cleared, and so on — but I had not stepped forward to advocate for New Hampshire children in need. Perhaps I had been too frightened, perhaps I had been too self-involved, but I recalled my breathlessness when I spoke to the Warren sixth-grade class, and I could not talk myself into becoming involved in the hurly-burly of abusive parents, court cases, children with profound disabilities, and all the rest of our social injuries.

Nevertheless, I did not immediately respond to the volunteer coordinator. I held on to her email asking me for my status, stalled by the meaning of her request. In short, it was time to step off the seesaw. I could not kid myself that someday I would bounce back and take up my position in CASA. For that matter, I could not persuade myself that I would ever have a chance to do productive work again. Occasionally friends or family might nudge me and ask what I planned to do in my retirement, but when they did I felt a contemptuous reply rise in my throat.

*I'm planning to die in retirement, that's what I'm doing*, I answered in my head. *That's my whole plan.*

It was an unfair response to a well-meaning question. What they wanted to ask, however indelicately, was *What now?* It was a question I knew too well; it was one I often asked myself. It was one thing to make calendar-filling appointments, to mark time by fishing trips, but they were asking a larger question.

What do you do now, buddy? What's a worthwhile endeavor to fill your remaining days?

The frank answer was, I didn't know. Time passed easily enough in the swirl of pills and appointments and new CT scans. My occupation, to a large degree, was being sick. I didn't like that. But was it realistic to look at sailboats, as I sometimes did, despite not knowing the first thing about sailing? To consider teaching a class at U Maine Machias? To follow my plan with Susan of building a small house on the land by the lovely estuary in Maine?

Saying *sorry, no thanks* to the volunteer coordinator at CASA acknowledged the final limits of my situation. My working life was done; my usefulness to society was finished. I could not even — as one local retiree in my town did — pick up trash on a daily walk. It was possible I was being too easy on myself, but I didn't think so. No matter how good I felt, and I felt pretty great at this point, all things considered, I couldn't ignore my need to stop to regain my breath after walking up a flight of stairs, or sweeping a floor, or doing the dishes.

Death had disappointed me. I felt like the child whose father says he will take him to the county fair, just hold on a second, he'd be right with me, but then never manages to get into the car. Death had offered me a ride, one I accepted reluctantly, and now I waited for him to put his keys in his pocket and slide into some moccasins. It may be a weak analogy, but it seemed I couldn't go out and play with friends, or make other plans to spend the day, because my father still might make good on his offer, might load me into the car and promise me cotton candy, might drive with one hand on the wheel, his elbow out the driver's-side window.

# 14

Susan moved in for a week and the weather snapped cold again. We spent our days beside the woodstove. Someone once called winter the season of cups and spoons, and that was certainly accurate to our experience. We ate her homemade chicken soup, drank tea, and worked in quiet communion. Most days she sequestered herself in an upstairs bedroom and spent the working day on Zoom with her office colleagues. I liked catching snippets of her voice throughout the day. I knew she could be talking to anyone from around the world or from some small town in New Hampshire. During breaks she came downstairs and sat by the fire and I rubbed her feet.

After dinner we fell into the habit of watching *Jeopardy!* and *Wheel of Fortune*. Television is the last thing in the world to interest Susan; she had not owned a television in her adult life, and her children were raised without it. But I subscribed to cable for the sports programming, primarily, although I was not immune from watching garbage TV. In any case, the game-show hour — seven to eight on the East Coast — became a little ritual we indulged in as we cleaned up the kitchen.

She was killer at *Wheel of Fortune*, often announcing the answers while I was still piecing together the smaller words. Afterward she usually took a bath while I fixed coffee for the morning and heated the kettle for the water bottle. We had once formed plans to hide out from winter somewhere down south, probably in one of the Carolinas, but my condition, coupled with the expanded Covid threats, persuaded us we were better off at home. We *cooped up*, as New Hampshire people call the art of staying warm and tidy in winter. A drop in temperature merely called for more wood in the stove.

It's a cliché to say it, but we slept like bears when we went to bed. Or like woodchucks, who are true hibernators unlike the somewhat restless bears. Deep under our covers, the winter wind chafing the windows and blowing snow across the meadow behind my house, we were warm and safe and happy. At first light we made coffee and then sat close to each other, our backs against the headboard, the pillows ample, and watched light come across the world while birds landed on a nearby crab apple tree to pick at the desiccated fruit that hung like brown pearls on the winter branches.

Not excitement, but deep, consoling comfort.

And we laughed. It would be difficult to explain what made us laugh, but we did. We did not laugh at people, or even situations. Mostly we found humor in the tangled wordplay that we shared between us. We even started a glossary, so that our pet words and puns could be documented and called back further down the road. Then a second cup of coffee, more dawn light, and gradually the call of the day to get back to work.

We were about four or five days into this pattern when Susan invited me to join her family on Zoom to celebrate her father's ninety-first birthday. I said yes at once, although I did not know her extended family intimately. I liked her father, Jim, immensely. He was born in 1931 and grew up in Chicago where his family owned a haberdashery. His mother had been a milliner and designer — it's hard not to love the words associated with this time and industry — but when women stopped customarily wearing hats and the factory closed, she landed a contract making pink floppy ears for Playboy bunnies. Jim's stories evoked a life of city bowling alleys, immigrant tailors, and Depression-era economics. Jim attended Notre Dame at his father's suggestion. He bowled for Notre Dame and worked in his father's store, where he was once held up at gunpoint. He went to all the home football games and even traveled back to South Bend on football weekends.

The Zoom birthday celebration was scheduled for five thirty. Susan dialed us in right on the button. We stayed close to the stove and greeted people as they popped into the Zoom screen. I wished Jim a happy birthday. Everyone did.

I come from a big family, but we do not get together on Zoom. I'm not sure why. But Susan's family was spectacularly represented. Her siblings, and their children, sat grouped around their respective cameras, all of them waiting for one another to speak. The younger children, some in high school, others in college, came in and said hello, wished their grandfather a happy birthday, then hung around, listening and watching, as one person after another told Jim they loved him.

How simple. How pure. How sublime.

I watched him closely. I admired him more than I can say. Who gets this rare gift at the age of ninety-one? His sons told him they loved him and tried to model their lives after him. Susan said much the same thing. They remarked on his patience, his kindness, his calmness. He had worked years at Xerox and IBM, had attended law school in his sixties, and had a second career as a university provost. He had always supported his children, had sent five kids through college, and now they turned to him and said he was the center of everything they knew or cared about. His granddaughter Chloe, who had just woken from sleep because as a first-year nurse she had a bunch of night shifts behind her, said that in her professional life — new and so wonderful — she had learned from her grandfather the tools and attitude that influenced her every day. She told him she loved him, admired him, kept him in mind whenever she faced a decision. Then another grandchild spoke through a garbled transmission — she was in Boston in a parking garage leaving work — that she couldn't wait to see him, that she loved him, and that she hoped he had the wonderful day he deserved.

Everything was love. Everything was offered to him in some small return for everything he had given them.

I held Susan's hand throughout the Zoom call. When we signed off, after singing happy birthday, after inquiring about the cake his other daughter, Megan, had made for his birthday, after saying goodbye to her brothers and their families, we sat for a long moment without saying anything. If beauty is the antidote to death, as it was in "The Emperor's Nightingale," then we had just seen true beauty. After a little while I told Susan that seeing that exchange, that family love, had been a privilege. She looked at me, a little surprised, then she nodded.

Sometime during that week, and several times before, Susan renewed a request that I make a list of books that had been important to me. Without being morbid, she thought it might bring her comfort to read some things I loved after I was gone. She thought it might be a way to have a conversation with me, of a sort. I worried that it could be dreary, but she assured me it wouldn't be for her and she promised to drop a book if it seemed to lead her in a lousy direction. She also pointed out that I often said I had lived as deeply in books and stories as I had in every-day life, which was true. Besides, I have always been a booster of books in a kind of emphatic way. I'm the guy who uses the word *must* a little too often when he suggests a read or a movie.

"Have you read *In Cold Blood*?" I might ask a friend or acquaintance or student. "Not the movie, not any of the movies, but the book? Oh, you must!"

I came by the habit honestly. Long ago in the American International School in Vienna, a friend, colleague, and fellow novelist, Jonathan Carroll (*Land of Laughs* and *Bathing the Lion* among many more), kept a shelf of books above his desk. Students knew he would take a reading of their character and interests, then reach forward and pluck a book out and hand to them a volume that he thought might be appropriately matched to their interests. He was famous for it; he was almost like an apothecarist. He offered only good reads, exciting works, that met the student where he or she currently stood. It was an inspired form of teaching on various levels. Not only did it often get a reluctant reader to read, but it told the student that he, Jon Carroll, was paying attention, that he cared enough to give thought to what the student might find interesting, while also opening up a conversation that could lead in a hundred beneficial directions.

I adopted the technique. Throughout my teaching career I had recommended books freely, trying to match, as Jon had done, a student's interest to a book that might engage or enlarge their world, might show some possibility that the student, in their youth, had only glimpsed. Often the recommendation fell on deaf ears, or ears not ready to hear what I offered, but occasionally I was surprised and delighted by the response. I recall handing a copy of Frederick Exley's astonishing *A Fan's Notes* — by no means a book everyone would enjoy — to a young man struggling to find his feet in college. He thanked me and dropped the book in his bag. Summer arrived and I never heard what he thought of the book, or if he had even attempted it, until I ran into him years later at reunion when he cornered me and told me that that book had found him at exactly the right time and space in his life. That had been my guess, and I took no special pride in its success; the book had done the work. I had merely been a matchmaker. Others have said, and I agree, that meeting someone who has read many of the same books as you have read is like meeting someone who has traveled to the same lands. I had been a troubled student in my day, and the irreverent, profoundly funny Exley voice would have been a tonic to me as an undergrad. I suspected that the student who had benefited by Exley was headed to the same land as I had visited, and the book served as a map to take him there.

So Susan had a point. Maybe a book would let us share some land even after I was gone.

But lists are impossible, as I tried to tell her. Books lead to books as surely as streams lead to rivers. Any list I could devise would necessarily fail or fall grievously short. It's like trying to say what is the best flower or tree. The best song. The prettiest ocean. I've always mistrusted literary awards on that count.

I compromised. I told Susan I would pretend to be a student coming to see my teacher self, decade by decade, to ask what book might speak to him. These were the books, I said, that had shaped me, which is a different thing from what I, as a pensioner and retired professor, consider the best books. I was also aware that my recommendations would reflect, and be limited by, my gender, age, and race. That was largely the point of the exercise.

I also refused to explain the reasons for the recommendations. That would be impossible. These were books that counted for me; I didn't promise, nor even expect, they would be of value to anyone else. I searched my memory for books that lingered in my mind, books that spoke to me in a time and place along the way. Finally, I told her I would skip books that might have influenced me as a child, as important as I believed them to be, and restricted my list from adolescence onward.

It proved to be an absorbing homework assignment. I tried to do it without referring to any 100 Best lists or anything of the sort. If I was to be the semester-long course of study, this list, I reasoned, was the syllabus. I also made a decision not to use authors' names, because looking for a title, like using an old library card catalog, would lead Susan, or anyone else, into other books by the same author. It came out like this:

**Teens:** *Lord of the Rings; Treasure Island; Invisible Man; On the Road; Catch-22; Cat's Cradle; Look Homeward, Angel; One Flew Over the Cuckoo's Nest; Dracula; Jaws; The Source; Call of the Wild; QB VII; Bambi.*

**Twenties:** *Leaves of Grass, Watership Down, A Member of the Wedding, We Have Always Lived in the Castle, The Magus, Salem's Lot, Lonesome Dove, Cannery Row, The Godfather, Fear and Loathing in Las Vegas, The Odd Sea, The World According to Garp, Siddhartha.*

**Thirties:** *Rabbit Is Rich, The Golden Notebook, In Cold Blood, Crime and Punishment, The Last Boy, The Professional, Roots, Great Heart, Tropic of Cancer, King of the World, Judgment Ridge, Islands in the Stream, The Devil's Teeth.*

**Forties:** *The Islandman, Autobiography of Malcolm X, The Right Stuff, The Last Duel, War and Peace, The Orchard, The Secret History, Of Human Bondage, A River Runs Through It, Death Comes for the Archbishop, A Moveable Feast, We Took to the Woods, Nine Mile Bridge, A Fine Balance.*

**Fifties:** *Miriam at Thirty-Four, The Hair of Harold Roux, The Horsemen, Give Me My Father's Body* (reissued in a revised and updated edition as *Minik*), *Endurance, As I Lay Dying, Snow Falling on Cedars, Emma, The Long Lavender Look, Shadow Divers, The Devil's Candy, Moriarty, The Last Place on Earth, The Power and the Glory.*

**Sixties:** *Bleak House; The Sound and the Fury; Catherine the Great; Last Train to Memphis; The Warmth of Other Suns; Guns, Germs, and Steel; Between Flops; Pretty-shield;* the Deptford Trilogy; *Plenty-coups; Catcher in the Rye; A Tree Grows in Brooklyn; Memoir of a Geisha; Years of Grace.*

That, I told Susan, was that.

I also explained that I deliberately left out some of the great nineteenth-century novels, immensely enjoyable ones, assuming she would find those on her own. Any Top Books list would provide dozens of them. Again, the books on my list were merely books that meant something to me.

The list-making impulse, once fed, almost ran away with me. Best places I've visited? Favorite beaches? Most memorable summer day? Compiling lists raised the question of how we occupy ourselves. What is important to us. It also raised the question of how long our wishes, our thoughts, our works, would endure after us. Susan might read and think of me as she moved through the books I recommended, but in time her life would fade. As I wrestled with this idea, I came across an Etruscan word, *saeculum*, which is a concept, or marker, of a temporal interval. Generally speaking, it is the span of time lived by the oldest person present. The day will come, for instance, when the last person to have fought in Vietnam will die. Who was the last person to remember the Battle of the Little Big Horn, not as an historically inaccurate Errol Flynn movie, but as a fierce, bloody war on the great plains of Montana? Who will remember when spats were commonly worn, or a car had to be cranked to start, or when the clank of an ice delivery man carrying a fifty-pound block in tongs brought merriment to the afternoon?

I wondered, then, what would be my *saeculum*. Or whom. I wondered what young nephew or niece's child, siphoned through the tunnel of time, would see a faded photograph of me and search their memories for my name.

*I think he was some sort of a great-uncle*, she or he will say. *I don't remember exactly. Look at his clothes!*

# 15

Susan and I kept an eye on the weather, and when February promised a weekend of milder temperatures, we decided to run up to the retired post office in Maine. We had been battered throughout New England by several harsh winter storms, and we agreed it made sense to go check on the structure. Besides, we had been locked down because of Covid, and as we could pack all the food we would need, reducing our contact with people and potential infection, we couldn't find any reason not to go. We both needed to stretch our legs.

The only obstacle, actually, was the snow itself, which would cover the land and small driveway, making it difficult to park our car without getting stuck. I phoned a lobsterman I knew in the area, and he volunteered to plow a swipe near the road that we could use to park. He also promised to bring us a scallop feast, fresh off the draggers whose season ran from January into the middle of February. So early one Friday morning, shortly before Valentine's Day, we drove north and east and found ourselves skirting the waterline through Belfast and Ellsworth, Jonesboro and Machias.

It felt good. It felt normal, or B-T, as we sometimes called it. Before-Tagrisso. Except for the occasional breathlessness I experienced, I was reasonably fit. As we traveled, Susan pointed out landmarks we had collected together, or ones she knew from her trips up to visit one of her daughters at the College of the Atlantic. We didn't listen to the radio; we didn't need to because our conversation never faltered. I sometimes worried that we tried to fit as much as possible into our times together because of the uncertainty of our future, but whatever the cause, we talked and laughed and held hands. We even rolled back the moonroof and enjoyed the pale February sun sawing into the top of our car. We wanted to smell the sea air, and we did.

The tiny post office is located on a beautiful road that runs up the northern edge of Leighton Neck, a peninsula that fingers into Cobscook Bay. It's always a moment for us when we pull onto the road, because shortly thereafter the land gives way to stunning water views. We try to guess where the tide will be; Pennamaquan Bay (it's also called Long Bay and sometimes the Pennamaquan River) is part of the great tidal wash most keenly felt in the Bay of Fundy. At low tide the entire perimeter of the bay drops to a muddy rib cage of sand and rockweed, then fills again until the water tries to climb the shoreline. Anyhow, it's a game we play before our arrival to guess at the stage of the tide, and on this trip we struck a falling tide, one that had just begun to pull the inland waters out to sea.

We concentrated so much on the water, and on whatever change had come to our cherished road, that we failed to notice at first the yellow tape that the police, apparently, had strung around a house across the road from us. Once we spotted it, I slowed down and we both rubbernecked to see what had happened. We knew the house, of course; it was the closest house to us, and it was notable for the vast pile of garbage that had been placed in the back of a disabled pickup parked permanently near the front porch. We also knew the house because of the owner's dog, a forlorn-looking brindled Staffordshire terrier, fairly young, we thought, who sat chained to the front staircase through long afternoons. The whole setup was a classic testament to rural poverty, and so we were not entirely surprised to see that something had occurred.

"That's a crime scene," Susan said, turning her head to catch one more glimpse before we turned onto the plowed scrape our lobsterman friend had made for us. "Something happened here. They don't put up yellow tape for no reason."

"Well, we'll find out soon enough."

But first we had to transport our bags and camping gear across an acre of ice and shin-deep snow. I had packed one of those plastic, drag-behind sleds that are popular with ice fishermen. We pulled it out of the car and loaded it, but Susan wouldn't hear of me pulling it. She worried that I would be overmatched or fall. I didn't fight her over it. When we were ready, we trudged down the incline to our miniature house, happy, as we always were, to arrive at our favorite place in the world. Then more rituals: we rang the marine bell three times to say hello, greeted our cement statue of St. Francis waiting for us on the deck, then opened the door. We had selected our day for fair weather, and the house, with all its windows, held enough heat and sunlight to make it comfortable inside, about sixty degrees. We wedged the door open and unloaded the sled. We made the bed, started a fire in our stove, then stood for a little while on the deck counting the boats in the scallop fleet. We made it as fifteen boats, although whether all were dedicated scallop fishers was hard to determine. The boats swung to face the tide: on a falling tide their bows pointed inland, at a rising tide, they pointed to the larger sea.

As we settled in, I texted our lobsterman friend and asked him about the scallops and about the yellow tape around the neighbor's house. He answered right away because, evidently, this yellow-tape incident was big news along our road.

Woman was killed Wednesday night. Drug deal of
some sort. Homicide.

I wrote back and asked what else he knew, but the event had
happened too recently and the echo was too new. Nevertheless,
the news stopped us for a moment. I couldn't help being
reminded that we — Susan and I — had ridden north on a wave
of privilege, that we came to vacation in a place where our neigh-
bors were sometimes desperate. I had experienced that same
feeling in beach locations around the world, in Indonesia or
Jamaica, Morocco or the Ivory Coast. Heaven knows we were
not ostentatious; we did not arrive on a yacht and spend the day
Jet Skiing up and down the bay. We could not afford anything
close to such opulence. But we had come north to have a cozy
weekend in a small cottage beside the water, to occupy ourselves
reading and painting, while nearby a neighbor we had never met
had felt she needed to sell drugs to survive.

Or maybe she had been an addict. Or maybe she made a
choice to dabble in criminality to make ends meet. Or maybe,
for all we knew, she ran a thriving business, pocketing huge sums
of money, while deliberately keeping a low profile.

That hardly seemed the case, but it was nonetheless a vexing
moral question, one we couldn't fairly approach without more
knowledge. We did, therefore, what most of us do in life — we
let it go, consigning it to the perpetual revisit-file we all carried
with us as humans. If I were honest, I couldn't say I had been
eager to meet our neighbor; her death did not change that
central fact. When we came up to Maine, we kept mostly to
ourselves; that was the object, really. Besides, the neighbor's
house looked ill kept and the garbage was piled high. The dog,
sadly, looked as if he could be aggressive if given the opportunity.
I wanted to be better, kinder in my appraisals, but there it was.

The idealism of youth had long ago been eroded into the bedrock of practicality.

It bothered me. It bothered Susan. Our presence on the land could not have been more benign. We deliberately kept ourselves out of local politics. The summer before we had been approached by a rockweed advocate. The woman who knocked on our door fought against the Canadian companies that came down our bay and cut rockweed that they would sell as fertilizer. She argued, environmentally, that the rockweed was necessary for periwinkle habitat, and for migrating birds, and she wanted us to take a stand with our beachfront to hold the line against the invaders. She was correct on all counts, I was certain, except that the local folks hired on to cut the rockweed made a few bucks to carry them through the fall. Did we — the woman asked — come down on the side of conservation? Then she mentioned that the local crews mooned her when they harvested near her property, hating her zealotry, and I realized, right or wrong, I had no sword to pick up in that particular fight.

What was our responsibility, then? How do we manage our lives while also trying to be fair and just to the people around us? How far do we go to influence the world? And how do we preserve our own small corner in it?

They were old questions, ones that I had discussed as a Peace Corps volunteer in the 1970s. Were we right to be in Africa? we had asked one another. Was our posting in a foreign culture warranted, especially given the legacy of European colonialism? Was it defensible to withhold aid if the consequence was death or famine? Regardless of how well intentioned we volunteers might be, were we unwittingly proselytizing for American culture and technology? The situation with our neighbor in Maine was not precisely analogous, but it rang some of the same bells of responsibility versus self-interest.

Susan and I talked about it while we made dinner, poured wine, and sat close to the stove. The temperature dropped. We were both tired. The beautiful evening light found the blue in the late-winter snow. A three-quarter moon stood high in the sky. A forceful breeze hit the side of the building now and then and brought out a low-throated whine.

Before bed, Susan checked on her phone and discovered a news release that appeared in the *Bangor Daily News*.

PEMBROKE, Maine — The death of a 53-year-old Pembroke woman was ruled a homicide this week, officials say.

A news release from Maine Department of Public Safety spokeswoman Shannon Moss stated Kayla Mead [not her real name] was found dead on Wednesday evening. The Washington County Sheriff's Office responded to 515 Leighton Point Rd. for a report of an unresponsive woman, according to Moss.

"Maine State Police Major Crimes Unit North and the Maine State Police Evidence Response Team responded to the residence to continue to investigate the circumstances surrounding her death. The victim was later transported to the Office of the Chief Medical Examiner in Augusta, where an autopsy was performed on Thursday, February 10, 2022," the release stated.

The autopsy results ruled the death to be a homicide.

Anyone with information about the death or who saw anything suspicious on Leighton Point Road in the last few days is asked to call Maine State Police in Bangor at 207-973-3700 and leave a message for Det. Adam Bell.

It didn't include anything about drugs, but perhaps our lobsterman friend knew something that was kept out of the paper for the time being. We let it go. After we refilled the coal stove one more time, then blew out the kerosene lanterns, we lay for a long time in silence.

"I wonder what happened to the dog," one of us said.

In the morning, at first light, Susan made us cowboy coffee — hot water through a filter over a carafe — while I worked on the coal stove. A few weeks before I had come across a song in an old movie and I had memorized the first two verses. It was sung with a happy, lively rhythm, nearly a shanty, so I serenaded Susan.

> *This is the day we give babies away*
> *With a half a pound of tea*
> *You just open the lid, and out pops the kid*
> *With a twelve month guarantee.*
>
> *This is the day we give babies away*
> *With a half a pound of tea*
> *If you know any ladies who want any babies*
> *Just send them round to me.*

I had never heard of it before, but I had discovered it was a reasonably well-known folk song and had appeared in two movies along the way. It was also a little jingle to sing to a cranky child, because the rhythm and rhyme created a perfect rocking cadence. I sang it until Susan begged me to stop, then we climbed back into bed and watched the sun come to find us.

Perhaps because of the murder across the way from us, we got on the topic of regrets. It was a topic that interested me keenly, because I had discovered one of the appealing features of my cancer diagnosis was the notion that soon, before long, any regrets I had piled up over a lifetime would disappear. We concentrate so sharply on the good we will lose by dying that it's easy to ignore the fact that our slates, for better or worse, will be washed clean at our death. If one were a notorious murderer, I suppose, that might not be the case, but the small sins and misdeeds of the average woman or man would rapidly fade from memory. I found that consoling, but when I said that to Susan, she looked mildly shocked.

"Do you have a lot of regrets?" she asked. "What kind of regrets?"

"Oh, small transgressions. I should have been a vegetarian all these years. That was simple laziness on my part."

She laughed, but she repeated the question.

What were my regrets?

I couldn't answer the question right away, which made me realize I needed to give it more thought. It also made me understand she had hit on something that pained me to think about. When I turned the question on Susan, she admitted she had a few regrets, but none that were particularly grave. She had let a few friends drift away; she had sometimes been cross with her ex-husband. She had made some goofs in her dating life, and she maybe allowed herself to be guided into a field of study, and college, because she had not known what was truly available to her. That's what it meant to be a woman in a certain culture at a certain time and that was a regret that had not been of her doing. Still, it nibbled at edges of her life.

For my part, I found myself focused on social interactions that had not gone well. I had been a rude know-it-all at times, an argumentative jackass who tried to make a dull evening into something exciting when it clearly was not the vibe everyone else felt. Some of it had to do with drinking and the false courage that went with it. Some of it had to do with boredom. Dating girls as a young man, I had never been purposely cruel, but I had been in a hurry of some sort, without understanding why, or what for, and my profound ignorance and impatience worked against me. I had also flopped a few times while giving a talk or speech, once quite memorably, and I was glad to think of those recollections going away.

I was sufficiently inculcated with boyhood Catholicism that I could divide my sins into mortal and venal, sins of commission and sins of omission. I wondered, frankly, what most people lived with in terms of regret. Was I average? I couldn't remember doing anything too baldly reprehensible, but, of course, that was from my standpoint. Perhaps some people, hearing I had passed away, might mutter for the devil to take me.

I had been divorced twice. Joking with buddies, I had called the marriages World War I and World War II, but that was an attempt to get a cheap laugh. I had been sincere in both marriages, each time certain I had gotten it right. Each marriage lasted thirteen years, almost as if I had an expiration date stamped on my kneecap. I regretted the pain and trouble I certainly caused those women. I had not meant to hurt anyone, and I was a good spouse in many ways, but the fact remained that, try as we might, we had not stayed together. That pain lingered in the world. Occasionally I wondered if I should have done something differently, tried harder, been kinder, more sympathetic, been less the ten-year-old, glib, competitive brat who had been formed, like some damn igneous rock in the volcano of Irish Catholic life, as the youngest child in a large family.

I would be glad to be shut of those memories. They could not haunt me much longer. I understood they were part of living, part of trying to make a full life, and I did my best to forgive myself. My regrets were not inert, however; they were a thick cauldron set above an unknowable flame that caused different moments of anguish to float to the top of the broth in painful bursts. Most of my regrets I would have forgiven in a stranger without a thought, but I knew myself, knew what I was capable of carrying out, and those stirrings of self-knowledge came late at night and in the early glimmering daylight.

I could have done more for people. That was my sin of omission. I had been selfish in the pursuit of my own life, my own desires. Yes, I had been a teacher, and I had done my duty as an educator, but I could have done more. It was not my nature to run for office or serve on boards, but I could have devoted time to the betterment of my community. And I was not kidding when I told Susan I should have been a vegetarian. I had, in fact, been one for three years sometime in my forties, but I had drifted away from it, lured by bacon, until I was once again a full-fledged flesh eater. I knew better; I could not plead ignorance about the treatment of animals that had died for my consumption. My inherent laziness, my shrugging-shoulders way, had given me permission to indulge myself. It was a trait I did not honor in myself.

I knew as a novelist that we remember the criticisms of our works long after forgetting the praise people lavished on them. Tell me a fault in my book and you have my attention; compliment it and I blush and try to get away. It was much the same in reviewing my journey. I had been courageous at times; I had once saved a life. I had always had an open hand, stood my fair share of drinks, had liked to laugh, had not carried vengeance with me, had adored children and pets, had been solicitous of the weak and infirm, had held doors and pulled out chairs, respected the elderly, paid my taxes, been a humorous uncle, and so on. What was laudable, however, seemed cheap currency.

Most men or women would have done as much. But my sins, large or small, were reserved especially for my private consumption. The good could be remembered by someone else; the bad was my own special worry stone.

So that would be over someday in the not-too-distant future.

Meanwhile, we had porcupine problems. Porcupines liked the old post office. I knew from reading about them that they were drawn to salt in the wood, but I had trouble imagining what salt remained in lumber that was a century old. As cute as they were — and they were very cute — they are notorious pests around cabins and ski lifts. We had not been asleep very long on our second night when we heard the grinding cadence of a porcupine gnawing at the side of the house. It was a steady, consequential sound. I stood up beside the bed and stamped several times, thinking that might chase him off, but he did not even bother stopping to catch a breath. A porcupine did not have to run or escape. It carried its defense with it at all times.

"We need to put some chicken wire around the bottom of this place," I said, probably for the tenth time. "He'll eat right through the building."

"How do you get rid of them?"

"I don't honestly know. Trap them, I guess. Or shoot them."

"Would you shoot one?"

"How much of the cottage is it going to eat?"

Perhaps another reward of cancer: I did not have to wage a porcupine war.

It was cold and quiet in the morning. The small warm spell we had anticipated had gradually begun to slip away to the east. I loaded the stove one more time so that we would be warm as we packed, then we reversed the rituals of arrival. Three bells to signal our departure, a handshake with St. Francis, then Susan pulled the sled up to the car.

Police cars surrounded the house of yellow tape. Because it was a Sunday, the police who worked the scene appeared casually dressed. It struck me again how two sets of lives — Susan's and mine with the woman who had been murdered — could approach each other so closely yet remain on different tracks. From my standpoint, I had been involved with my illness and trying to understand what it meant to be dying. This woman, this Kayla Mead, had somehow found her way to a house only a few hundred yards from ours, had done what she needed to do to survive, and then had been killed by someone who either required the drugs she offered or had little regard for life. I wondered if she had experienced a moment of peace once she had accepted her fate. I hoped so. Standing by the car, everything felt tied together: the woman's death, my illness, the young woman in the Portsmouth hospital who had attempted to end her life, even the porcupine, craving salt, who funneled his rodent teeth along the lumber formed from trees harvested more than a century ago. It mixed me up. Everything felt transitory and beautiful, craven and sublime. The earth felt hungry, as if it could not be satisfied by people remaining above the soil. Entropy is the natural state of the world, I knew, and that to stand erect, to move about the earth, is the rare, exceptional thing. When we climbed in the car and pulled away, we saw the police standing in small pockets around Kayla Mead's front yard, her door open, the yellow tape already sagging onto the grass.

# 16

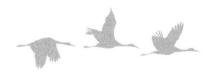

With winter slowly backing off, I got in the habit of reading in my woodshed. I had built the shed myself, and while I am not much of a builder, I at least had the foresight to face the shed opening to the south, so that the sun, in all seasons, could bake the cordwood needed for us to live in New Hampshire. In the early afternoon, I carried my books and magazines out to the shed, plopped down in a lawn chair, and took as much sun as possible in the growing spring light. Out of the wind, I read and dozed, my waking sometimes comical — Where was I? What was happening? — and sometimes as calm as a great reptile slowly lifting its eyes above the water sheen. I read a Raymond Chandler novel, *Farewell, My Lovely*, and didn't like it much, although I saw his gift for simile. I read a Robert Parker novel, *Melancholy Baby*, tried Daphne du Maurier's *House on the Strand*, read one hundred pages of a novel recommended by a friend and couldn't get into it. I read long articles in *The New Yorker*, a few short stories, the last two books of the Deptford Trilogy, the better part of a nonfiction work on seahorses, and, in preparation for our trip out to see the sandhill cranes, a gift picture book Susan had sent me called *On Ancient Wings*. I liked sitting in the sun with the book open on my lap, pictures of cranes leaping about to court and squabble, while the sun slid behind my barn and substituted shadow for light.

Tired and cold by late afternoon, I returned to the house and fixed myself a scotch, sometimes two, and loaded the woodstove for another night of single-digit temperatures.

Part of me, on these lovely afternoons, wondered if this is how one died. Maybe it was wrong, I reasoned, to think of death as a single event. Maybe it was the accumulation of many days sitting in the sun, or naps under a heavy down comforter, or cups of tea. Maybe it was something that took place while you weren't paying attention, and my foolish attempt to monitor it, to *understand it*, was the most laughable of human preoccupations. Maybe it was the worst sort of vanity to think that we could pinpoint a moment and call that death. I had even read that one should draw a distinction between the illness that brings about death, and death itself. As cold is nothing more than the absence of heat, so death is simply the absence of life. Put accurately, it is the disease that takes us, usually with the aid of a heart attack or limitation of air, not death at all. I envied the animals, who lived, as far as we know, without a sense of their own mortality. On the occasions when I had gone to the vet to have a dog euthanized, I had always found it remarkable that the beloved creature could not divine that I was a Judas bringing her or him to a final moment. Then the doctor, then the syringe, then the slow, merciful breath of parting.

Meanwhile, with a stronger sun combined with freezing temperatures at night, my driveway turned into a sheet of ice. If I had been thirty years old, I probably wouldn't have noticed, but now — so much like the older man in Katherine Mansfield's "Her First Ball" who predicts the protagonist will someday dread the dance floor due to its slipperiness — I could not take the short walk to my vehicle without feeling absurdly vulnerable and fragile. I was not an old, old man, I didn't think, but I was an ill old man, one who could sustain serious injury if he fell. I took to leaving a pair of decrepit boots with creepers attached to the soles beside the door so that I could walk confidently to get the mail. How humbling. How necessary. How easily unforeseen when we are young.

Susan came for a visit and we cut crab apple wands and brought them inside to force. I've never had much luck with forcing things, but Susan said we had to have hope and, remarkably, in two weeks' time small green buds appeared on the branches. The root water turned brown with tannins, and small tendrils of growth searched at the bottom of the vase for soil. The seasons were turning; spring was a mere three weeks away. On my drives to the grocery store, I spotted sap buckets hung on the sugar maples. And one evening, just at sunset, I heard a phoebe's unmistakable call announcing its return to the northern forests.

A strange thing happened the night after Susan went home. I woke in the deepest part of the night to the sound of music playing. Because I knew I was alone in the house, I came fully awake, just on the calm side of full alarm. Nothing like it had ever happened before in the two-plus decades I had lived in the house. It took a moment to realize the music was not electronic; it was not the product of a computer suddenly coming on, the mouse nudged by an actual mouse, perhaps, but something higher and more childlike. I knew the score of a horror movie when I heard one, and this tinkling tune certainly qualified as the beginning of one. My body flushed with adrenaline. A sardonic, mocking part of my brain asked if my time had come, if this was not the sound of angels coming to fetch me! Then, little by little — the house dark as the interior of an old camera — I realized the sound came from my mother's ancient jewelry box, a somewhat silly little airport gift my father brought home from a trip of some sort probably a half century before. When my parents died and our house sold many years ago, I had asked to have the box, because I remembered as a small boy winding it and playing it while my mother dressed to go out to dinner. I knew the tune down to every note. And here it was, in the middle of the night, choosing this moment to play its somewhat ghostly score.

I waited for a long moment, listening. Then I turned on my light and picked up the jewelry box. I could not recall winding it recently; it was not something I often looked at or even bothered with. Holding it on my lap, I lifted the lid and got the tune to play more forcefully. Then as quickly as it had started, it stopped. The explanation that slowly bloomed in my foggy mind made sense: Something in the room's temperature or atmospheric pressure had changed, and the final portion of my last winding had suddenly been released. Yes, it was an odd little event, one that, in Victorian times, might have inspired a séance, but in a modern light it triggered nothing as notable. It was easy to see, however, how such events could marshal in a dozen spurious explanations. Maybe my mother's spirit had come to visit! Any sort of ghost story would have done nicely.

On the last Friday in February, a lovely winter storm visited. Snow began in the morning and continued to fall all day, a light, beautiful snow that arrived without wind. I sat close to the woodstove and drank tea. As a teacher, I always appreciated a snow day, and this was clearly such a day. The radio buzzed with school and business closings and information about the duration of the storm and what depth the snow might reach. At three I went out and stood for a while in the back meadow, happy to breathe the winter scent, pleased to see a pair of priestly black crows perched in an aspen. I have long loved Wallace Stevens's "Thirteen Ways of Looking at a Blackbird" and I can even recite small pieces of it. Standing in the meadow, I remembered these lines:

*It was evening all afternoon.*
*It was snowing*
*And it was going to snow.*

The snow reached a foot before the plows came to take it. The trees held the snow on their branches as long as they could, and the next morning, in first light, everything began to melt and the sunshine found its reflections in pools and in water dripping from the roof.

On March 1, I sent off my taxes to a firm that had prepared my returns for twenty years. I've always been a terrible bookkeeper, and an absolute incompetent when it came to recording and managing receipts, but with the help of Christine, my wonderful accountant, I usually came up with something that at least didn't get me thrown in prison. Truthfully, I never minded paying taxes; I always felt it was our responsibility as citizens to pay our fair share, and, except when the taxes seemed to me to be spent in wasteful ways, usually in the execution of a foreign war, I was willing to do my part. As a writer, I am classified by the Internal Revenue Service as an independent contractor — like a self-employed electrician or a gig worker in a ballpark — which means the usual deductions are not taken from my pay stubs. Tax season always makes me nervous, as a result, and inevitably I feel like a perjurer by the end of April. It never fails to remind me of the Catholic confession I experienced as a boy, a sort of phony affair where you are supposed to enumerate all the sins, big and small, that you committed since the last session in the local confessional box. The priest never seemed to take seriously what I conjured out of thin air for the sake of polite conversation — I lied three times to my parents, was once cross with my sister, and stole a piece of Juicy Fruit from Doug Morash — and neither, I guessed, did the IRS.

But now I had medical bills, substantial ones, and I was unsure how or if the IRS credited these sums as deductions. Going through my checkbook, and then my Mastercard receipts, I wrote down the best guess I could at the cost of being sick.

**Medical Costs**
$5,250 for Tagrisso (cancer drug)
$42 Speare Memorial radiology
$362 Harvard Pilgrim
$20 Mid State Medical
$24.38 Radiology
$117.78 Radiology
$181 Harvard Pilgrim
$181 Harvard Pilgrim
$74.33 Portsmouth Hospital
$10 Mid State Medical
$181 Harvard Pilgrim
$181 Harvard
$181 Harvard
$181 Harvard
$181 Harvard
$25 CVS
$12 CVS
$17.38 CVS
$9.20 CVS
$22 Rite Aid N. Hampton
$133.86 AARP dental
$36.54 CVS
$29.28 CVS

By a rough calculation, adding just the dollars and not the cents, that came out to approximately $7,500, or $600 a month, more or less. That was with insurance. Actually, it was probably higher, because I did not have medical expenses throughout the year. The list represented the seven months since my diagnosis. It just so happened that I had gone off my medical plan at my retirement less than a week before the cancer diagnosis arrived. For a horrid moment at the end of May, I had been terrified that I was exposed completely, caught in a gap between my employer insurance and Medicare. Fortunately, after a little wiggle here and there, and with my son working the phones to make sure of my coverage, my insurance was widely accepted. I had to pay deductibles, of course, sometimes sizable ones, but I was under some sort of umbrella. What the shape and scope of that umbrella might be seemed to change at every appointment. Little was uniform, little was predictable. And naturally, I was expected to make all these arrangements while feeling the first wave of cancer cover me and reduce my strength. Luckily, I had help.

What did my nine months of cancer cost the system? What did the hospital charge the insurance companies? No idea, although I know it was astronomical. Occasionally I spotted something on a bill indicating that Medicare had covered a treatment, usually a CT scan or X-ray, that costs tens of thousands of dollars. It was indecipherable to me. Not only that, not once in nearly a year did I meet a fellow patient who knew what exactly was covered, what costs could be anticipated, what were the limits of their reach. Furthermore, I often found myself standing in front of a billing person who bashfully informed me that I owed money, or who had the unpleasant task of telling me this or that treatment had not been approved. Frequently I had to lay out any medical-related cards I owned on the desk between us to ask them to pick one that worked. I came to accept the grind of the process, rarely asking questions or batting an eye when a large bill arrived.

But according to a study I read, one in six people gives up treatment because she or he cannot afford it. Given a choice between bankruptcy or death, the individual chose death.

As I understood our country's 2017 tax policy shift, my costs, if not greater than the standard deduction allowable, would not be worth itemizing. I had never been good at calculating these types of percentage problems — thus the accounting firm — and I found the entire process confusing and vaguely humiliating. I had always paid my bills on time, but the health care system made such scrupulousness nearly impossible. It removed a portion of my dignity by turning me into a befuddled, somewhat cynical retiree who looked carefully at bills before abandoning any hope of full comprehension. It turned me into a stereotypical cranky old man, a figure of mockery in our culture, a person of no real worth.

From what had been asked of me financially, I had two remaining opinions about the whole ordeal of medical expenses. First, the billing and payment schedule for nearly everything I did was a hodgepodge, with some fees coming out of pocket X, others from pocket Y, and with few people able to navigate the overarching system competently. I certainly didn't understand it and couldn't pretend to. The second point was more positive: For all of its failing and confusion, I had weathered nearly a year of medical treatments without going broke or draining all of my savings. It had been an expense, certainly, and I was aware that I was privileged and fortunate to be able to meet the challenge set by sophisticated health care. Again, I wondered what happened in the lives of people without resources or the time and health needed to deal with these arcane matters. Supervising and keeping abreast of payments and billing could quickly evolve into a full-time occupation, and I could not imagine working steadily at a job while maintaining an appropriate financial ledger. Phone calls to insurance companies could take up the better part of a day before resolving a dispute or a misunderstanding. Often the claims and counterclaims melted into a Gordian knot, an unsolvable one, that seemed to be kicked down the road for future discussion.

When people asked, as they sometimes did, what I thought of our medical system now that I was squarely in it, I shifted the ground under the question and cited a paradigm Susan told me about the disability community with which she worked. She learned early in her educational training that people who are disabled call the able-bodied members of society *temps*. You know that ramp in front of your neighbor's house, she asked, or the wheelchair buttons inside the gym doors? Those modifications are waiting for you. Most of us need help in the end, she pointed out. It's what it means to be human.

Preaching a little about the one thing I took away from experience, I would say that we need to stop seeing health care — and all aspects of its cost — as something extra, something to be concerned about in the future, something that happens to someone else. I had been a *temp*, blindly so, and now my time had come. When I told the interlocuter my response to the health care system I always ended by saying, *You are not far behind, I promise.* The crutch, the ramp, the raised toilet will be yours someday, too. Like Ahab beckoning from the flank of the white whale, *all shall follow.*

# 17

I once spoke to a man who had been swept out to sea by a tsunami. He had been vacationing in Indonesia around Christmas 2004 when, unbeknownst to him, a 9.1 undersea earthquake occurred as two tectonic plates — the Australian and Indian Plates — collided off the coast of Sumatra Island. The collision of the plates resulted in a massive megathrust quake, a phenomenon that occurs when a heavy ocean plate pries under a lighter one. A nine-hundred-mile stretch of Pacific fault line fractured instantly, causing the ocean floor to rise abruptly by forty meters. Within twenty minutes of the earthquake a monstrous wave sped toward Banda Aceh, and when it landed it killed more than one hundred thousand people and turned the city to rubble. Subsequent waves, all reaching the height of approximately one hundred feet, landed on India, Thailand, and Sri Lanka. Eight hours later and five thousand miles from its Asian epicenter, the tsunami crashed into South Africa's coast, devouring its final victims.

The tsunamis, collectively, killed approximately 230,000 people in total, making it one of the world's largest modern-day disasters. It became known as the Boxing Day tsunami, because the events played out on December 26, the day after Christmas.

When the fellow told me about the tsunami — he was a man I worked with in publishing — he was still in acute shock about what had occurred. He was young and resilient, but nothing could have prepared him for a tidal wave crashing onto the beach where he was staying, thrusting everything inland, then, with a sickening turn, slowly drawing everything back toward the open ocean. The tongue of the water had attached to him, and it had tugged him underneath the incoming surface, nearly drowning him in the first moments of his ordeal, then gushed him out with the returning suck until he was well out to sea. He grabbed onto anything that floated and spent hours clinging to the detritus of an island resort community, his body rigid with shock, the water heaving, the possibility of sharks a potent, primitive danger.

"What I remember most," he told me, "is the still, sickening feeling I experienced when the water drew back. It does, you know? Before a wave of that magnitude arrives, it sucks everything toward it. The beach empties. All the lagoon and bay water disappears and suddenly you see parts of the beach you never expected to see. You see the actual sand. It almost feels like a joke. And when you look out to sea, at first you think something marvelous is happening. Then gradually you start to understand that something is coming toward you, something vast and deadly, and there is no time to run, really, no time to do much of anything."

He was saved, obviously, by a fishing boat sometime in the first evening. The fishing boat had to move with extreme caution for fear of crashing into large obstacles washed out to sea.

Maybe I am trying too hard to connect my situation with something more graphic, more dynamic, but I thought of this man's story often as I waited for my next medical appointment. The mental image of water drawing out, emptying into the maw of the rushing wave, seemed dreadful to me. When he had told me that at first he thought something wonderful and eventful was happening, I sympathized with him. Who, looking out on a quiet tropical evening, imagines that the placid scene before him will momentarily transform into an atrocious nightmare, with gray-white water carrying eight stories of waste and energy in a fist that will explode on the land? Who is wise enough to look at the retreating water seconds before the wave appears on the horizon and decipher its true meaning?

Too big a reach, perhaps. But it was, and continues to be, a metaphor that worked for me, that at least helps me visualize what has occurred in my life. I was going along happily, glad to be putting my teaching career behind me, when, suddenly, my breath grew shorter and a pain in my back grew more pronounced. The water sliding out to sea, in other words. I cannot kid myself that a wave is not forming out beyond my sight, perhaps beyond the horizon; I know it is there. The only thing to be determined is how big the wave might be and where it will strike land. There is little question of its capacity for devastation.

The trick is, I tell myself, to ignore the wave. Is that the right course of action? In the most basic way, we all must ignore the wave. But I realized as spring began to make vivid signs of its approach that I had been cowardly in surrendering to the wave. True, I had not fallen for the fake exhortations about fighting the good fight, or defeating cancer, but I had ceded ground to it that I needed now to recover.

Another metaphoric story.

Susan's daughter Ruthie used to be responsible for getting eggs from the family chicken coop. A nice, appropriately scaled job for a young person, unless, as often happens in rural New Hampshire, some predator has slipped in during the night and wreaked havoc among the hens. It happened frequently enough around Susan's homestead that Ruthie developed a somewhat cynical turn of mind about it.

"The chickens are dead," she always thought as she walked to the coop. "Any hens left living are a bonus."

It slowly dawned on me that I had done something similar regarding my health. I had assumed the tsunami was on top of me, that the chickens were dead — to mix metaphors hopelessly — when, in fact, I was still very much alive. I had become not despairing, but resigned. Instead of trying to eat nutritious meals, I let myself indulge any whim in terms of food. I did not exercise. I did not see the point of trying to improve my condition, because, in point of fact, the wave was coming to sweep it all away.

But then Susan's hairdresser, Basil, said he thought I would live at least a decade longer. Absurd! We had never met! Yet his simple proclamation, coming as it did without an effort to prove it true, somehow heartened me. Why couldn't I live ten more years? People had done it. Yes, the wave was large and forceful, but I had no guarantee the water had drawn all the way back. The wave could still be forming, the bowstring still being pulled taut. Why, I wondered, was I so willing to believe the worst outcome and not the best?

Without meaning to, or maybe for legitimate causes, I had put my life on pause. Permanent pause. Some of it was due to Covid, and to the impenetrable frigidity of a New Hampshire winter, but a more insidious element was the fatal resignation I had claimed for my own. Surely, I slowly reasoned, there was a middle ground. Surely there was a way to push forward boldly, while also recognizing that the clean beach was evidence of something mortal coming toward me. I needed to stop linking my feeling of good health, which was won for me by Tagrisso (but was real nonetheless), with the fateful day when the wave would come into view. After all, the suddenness of the original diagnosis was proof that we could not always know what was coming toward us. Hell, maybe Basil was right! Why not assume some of the hens were alive and contentedly producing eggs in their warm, cluck-filled coop?

To commemorate this change in paradigm, I bought a kite. Silly perhaps, but I used it as a symbol that I could still take pleasure in physical things. I forced myself to go for longer walks than I had heretofore attempted, and on one warm morning I rolled out my yoga mat and tried to go through a series of sun salutations. I was never very good at yoga, and never really disciplined about rolling out my mat, but it felt correct to resume a practice that I had put on hold.

*Hoping to cease not until death*, Whitman tells us in *Song of Myself*, and I wanted it to become my motto. He adds several stanzas later:

> *All goes onward and outward, nothing collapses,*
> *And to die is different from what any one supposed,*
> *and luckier.*

It made sense to assume more years; it was the only wager worth making. If I was wrong, cancer would correct me quickly enough. If I was right, however, I would derive the benefit of the assumption. I decided that my budding building career — at least as I dreamed it — could resume as well. I began sketching out a shed/office I wanted to build for Susan on our property in Maine and began plans for a tent platform where we could pitch a canvas tent in case people wanted to visit. Not exactly the Taj Mahal, I knew, but to put two boards together is a form of hope. And maybe a dog, I considered. Maybe I could let my heart go that far forward.

Just as I was trying to regain my balance regarding the future, Russia attacked Ukraine. We all know the story. A crazed despot wanted to re-annex what he considered part of his splintered nation, and, having sufficient military might to do it, he rolled his tanks toward the capital. Like most people witnessing this bald aggression, I had a variety of emotions: disgust with human cruelty, admiration for the Ukrainian citizens' bravery, despair at the ongoing need for humankind to wage war. In all ways, it was an old story. It was also a white, European story. During the past half decade, more than five million African children under five years of age had died and the world had been largely silent about it.

Still, the Ukraine siege was horrible to watch. The chief difference between this conflict and former conflicts was the presence of social media. This was, perhaps, the first war to be fought with a million cameras trained on the atrocities, a hundred thousand reporters ready to tell the rest of the world the conditions on the ground. I found it fascinating and sad. I found the conjectures about the despot's mental condition reductive — of course he was a madman, because who else but madmen think our time on earth should be spent bringing bloodshed to the world? I tried to imagine what it must be like to say to those listening for orders, *Now go, bomb your cousins, lay waste to cities, destroy whatever human harmony we have thus far achieved in the world.*

Some people just want to watch the world burn.

That line, I think, was from a Batman movie. Alfred tells Bruce Wayne a simple story about a brigand in Burma who robbed and murdered for no material gain. When Bruce Wayne looks puzzled, Alfred delivers the line about watching the world burn. You can't negotiate with a man like the Burmese brigand. He wants nothing, in the end, but the destruction of the world.

I actually thought the line appeared originally in a Graham Greene story called "The Destructors." In that disturbing British story, published in 1950, a teenage gang plots to break in and destroy, piece by piece, beam by beam, a two-century-old house owned by someone the boys label as Mr. Misery. They plan it for Mr. Misery's bank vacation week and, like termites, they eat the house from the inside out. There are a few plot bumps along the way, mostly about Mr. Misery returning early and being locked in the outhouse, but in the end a lorry driver assists the boys by hooking a rope to one of the house's pillars and yanking it down. Even the lorry driver laughs at the collapse of what was once a beautiful structure.

The error we inevitably make when watching something like the horrors of Russia's adventurism in Ukraine is to ascribe to it a rational basis. It is not rational. It's impossible to say the world, or even one's own country, becomes better by such aggression and killing. In the past, certainly, propaganda could persuade a population to go to war (it worked devastatingly well in our country, alas), but now those little phones in every hand reveal the lie. Destruction is not creative, as some defenders of the protagonist in "The Destructors" sometimes argue. Destruction is a thief and a coward. It thwarts progress; it invites regression.

Two events occurred, however, to distract me. First, a flock of cedar waxwings, returned from the southlands, landed on two crab apple trees visible from my bedroom. Cedar waxwings are dramatically colored, with a yellow, horizontal stripe on the tip of the tail and a black mask — like a child's Halloween mask — across their eyes. The adult males often have a red mark, just a spark, in the middle of their wings. They are acrobatic in their pursuit of berries and dried crab apples, often hanging upside down to get at the fruit. They arrive and feed in clusters, and where before cardinals and robins had come to pluck at the crab apples, the cedar waxwings did not mess around. In the course of two days, they cleaned the trees completely, like "The Destructors" themselves, though I understood they would transport the trees' seeds inside their bodies and distribute them throughout the county. Their beauty was a small, quiet answer to the ugliness of our violent world.

The second event occurred when a red squirrel snuck inside my house. It must have been the Houdini of red squirrels, because it appeared in the midst of cold days during an entire week when I had not had the doors opened except to pass quickly in and out. That meant, as I surmised, that the squirrel had access to some sort of hole or opening somewhere in the house or basement. What it did not mean, unfortunately, was that the squirrel remembered how to go out the way it had entered. For three days I had to steel myself for occasional squirrel sightings. Suddenly it would be implacably *there*, a classic squirrel silhouette sitting on its haunches regarding me. Now and then I heard it scamper across a floor, its sharp claws like dice rattling, then, as mysteriously as it arrived, it departed.

I was afraid of one thing particularly after receiving my diagnosis: that I would learn that I had caused my own cancer. I knew, naturally, that smoking was not good for a person and I had given it up well over thirty years before the initial radiology technician had blundered and asked me about a history of lung surgery. I had given it up precisely because I knew it could kill me. In fact, I had been walking up a hill shortly after I began teaching at Plymouth State University when I had to stop and catch my breath. The hill was legitimately steep, and people often lost their wind on the way up, but I recalled standing for a moment to rest and telling myself that I was much too young to be so winded. Besides being a dirty, addictive habit, I knew smoking could ruin one's lungs. I wasn't ignorant or naive. I didn't minimize the risk in my own thinking.

But I liked to smoke. It would be inaccurate, and somehow unfair to the young man who I was in those days, to say I didn't. I used to like to smoke while I wrote. I liked a cigarette with a glass of scotch. I liked coffee with cigarettes, and I can still remember the pleasure of a well-packed pipe with good tobacco, the invitation to loaf and sit still that a pipe brought with it. I smoked while I read. I enjoyed it. Asked why I smoked, I told people it was life's punctuation. Clean the basement, then have a smoke. Fix coffee, then a smoke. Some of the most vivid conversations I had in life took place with a fellow smoker, both of us dotting what we said by breaks to relight. I used to proclaim that I didn't trust anyone who hadn't smoked at some point in her or his life. In line with that behavior, it's safe to say I was never the student who sat at the front of the class and took copious notes. I was the hack-around fool at the back, taking it all with a huge wink and a nod, ready to be outside, to run and jump and climb and later, to smoke and drink and live! Smoking identified me — and others — as people who did not give too much of a good goddamn. We wanted a little bit of trouble, a little edginess in our days. I was young, in short, and filled with beans.

I also thought I was immortal. Indestructible. I had always had a strong constitution, one that earned me a football scholarship and a free college education. I wrestled and played baseball and became a pretty fair squash and handball player later in life. I learned how to hike and camp and fish while in my twenties. I carried heavy backpacks up mountains and rode bikes for miles. I was physical, in other words, with or without cigarettes. I could tough out most things if I set my mind to it.

I quit cold turkey on the day after New Year's Eve somewhere around 1990. I was strategic enough not to attempt to quit on New Year's Day, but on January 2, my brother Chuck's birthday, I put down all and any smoking devices and never picked anything up again. I had the usual difficulties in giving up nicotine, but once I pledged to do it, I held fast. Like many people, I suppose, I never thought cancer would result as long as I quit at a decent age. I was thirty-five, or thereabouts, and I was finished with tobacco. Who would guess that thirty years later cancer would knock on the door and ask if I remembered all those burning embers?

Quitting smoking reduces one's chance of cancer by half after ten to fifteen years. By twenty years it's reduced again. Nonetheless, one of the first questions the doctors and nurses asked me at Dartmouth was whether I had been a smoker. I didn't like answering that question or poring over statistics about smoking. If smoking was the cause of my cancer, and thereby an early death, so be it. I could as easily say I got cancer from being young and dumb. Besides, I rationalized that I had other risks. I had heated my house for three decades with wood and coal. Where were the stats on that risk? And what about food additives, asbestos in the cheap apartments I had rented, DDT sprayed to keep down suburban mosquitoes?

I assumed my answers around smoking fed into national statistics for some health survey somewhere. I didn't begrudge divulging the information, exactly, but I felt it was a little . . . rude. Would similar questions be put to someone who was overweight? Would an LNA somewhere, charged with taking down vitals of an obese patient, turn to them and ask, *When did you begin to eat eclairs?* Maybe so, but I doubted it. The plain and simple fact was that I had smoked, that I regretted it to a degree — it's very easy to regret once you get a lung cancer diagnosis — but that it fell, for me, into a wide range of youthful exploration and derring-do that could have landed me in terrible straits in any number of ways.

*So sue me*, as we used to say as kids.

But my tenderness and defensiveness around the question signified that I worried I had caused my own condition. Unforced error, as they say in tennis.

Meanwhile, my next appointment approached. Representatives from Dartmouth-Hitchcock called to confirm times and arrival plans, to give parking advice, and to confirm that my insurance carriers remained the same. Dr. Dragnev had ordered an MRI brain scan to make sure that my slight difficulty in word retrieval — and my dip in crossword and *Jeopardy!* competency — was not the result of the march of cancer. I was told not to eat the day of, then told I could eat the day of, then the question finally drifted away without anyone giving me a solid answer. I knew I had to absorb a contrasting dye, if not two, and so I decided to err on the side of caution and fast until midmorning, when the hard parts of the tests were squarely behind me.

As always, Susan made plans to come with me. She took a day off work and came up the night before to stay beside me. We had to wake at four forty-five to make the hour-and-a-half drive over to Dartmouth-Hitchcock. The sun came up as we drove, and Susan wondered if I was scared.

"I feel good," I said. "I don't think anything bad has happened. I think I would have felt it."

"Your face looks fuller, you know?"

"Do you mean fat?"

"No, fuller. Your cheeks were pulled in taut before."

"It will all be okay," I said, because I knew she had the slant of mind to dust every corner. It made her a superb instructor and a wonderful companion, yet it could also jam her up.

A little part of me, however, worried. I worried primarily about the brain scan. It would be rough, I figured, to be told that the cancer had advanced in my chest and other organs, but the brain was the tabernacle. If that went, the game was over. I had the image of it as a great, halved cabbage, the leaves on top standing in for my hair, the hemispheric line a vegetal cord, the white meat of the flesh the gray matter of my up-to-now-dependable brain. If cancerous blasts had colonized it — and I knew that they had — and had continued to grow despite Tagrisso, the world was about to become a dim place. It was possible, I knew, that Dr. Dragnev could step into the examination room and, with a downcast expression, explain that Tagrisso had at last been defeated and that cancer was again over the castle wall.

# 18

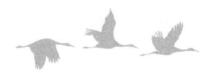

Joni Mitchell was a mistake.

I should hasten to add that I love and loved Joni Mitchell. She had been the author of a dozen powerful anthems while I was in college. It was impossible to walk through the dormitories on the Temple University campus during the early 1970s and not hear Joni belting out her soul-crushing sadness. Her magnificent album *Blue* colored the air, especially in girls' rooms, where she seemed a high priestess calling her fellow women *to be prepared to bleed*.

No, more accurately, it was *bleeeeeddddeeeed*. Soulful.

I found her music moving and wise and gorgeously composed. Nobody simply tossed a Joni album onto the turntable — yes, turntables then — and went about her or his daily tasks. Joni demanded attention. She wanted to tell you about *Richard [who] got married to a figure skater, and he bought her a dish washer and coffee percolator.* She wanted to draw a map of Canada, O Canadaaaaaa. With your name sketched on it twice!

I can still recite her lines, because one listened intensely to Joni. She was not background music, which was something I forgot when Brian, a burly MRI tech, asked if I wanted music while in the MRI tube. I only thought a moment before saying, "Joni Mitchell?"

"You got it," he said.

He asked this while he and a nurse slowly arranged me on the slide of the MRI machine. It was not even nine o'clock. I had had a blood draw already, a CT scan with a contrast dye that made me want to urinate, then had been waiting — in an absurd pajama outfit with huge pants, a backdoor johnny, and a knee-length terry robe — for an hour without a book, phone, or jigsaw puzzle. When I was finally called, my knees cracked loudly as I stood.

"Leave your locker key over there," Brian said, pointing to a windowsill once we were inside the machine room. "No metal, right? Did you ever work with metal?"

"No."

"Any surgeries, prosthetics, anything we should know about?"

"No, I think I'm clean," I said, reminded of airport security.

"Good deal. This should take about an hour and a half. And you have a port in your arm already?"

"I do. I got it for the CT scan."

"Terrific."

He unwrapped the gauze that had held the plastic port in place and folded it on my belly.

"That's the one thing I hate about the medical world," he said. "All the waste it generates."

"I can imagine," I replied, although I was mostly trying to work with the nurse to raise my knees, slide a pillow under my backside, and accept a hockey-mask contraption, complete with a rearview mirror, so that I would not feel claustrophobic in the tube.

"Surgery is even worse," Brian said, "they touch things once and they have to throw everything out. It's crazy."

"I bet."

By this time, I was properly positioned. It was not comfortable by a long shot, but I knew it was important not to move. Brian put a rubber ball in my hand that, he promised, would stop everything if I felt I needed it to stop. Then he pushed a button and I slid into the toaster.

Almost immediately the machine began to ping and clank and whir. Joni Mitchell came on at full volume. Earsplitting volume. And slightly off the station, or receiver, so that she sang through a gravel pit of static. I closed my eyes. I considered squeezing the rubber alarm bell, but we had only been under way less than a minute. That seemed a little precious on my part. I tried to relax into the music. Joni can be soothing and tranquil on occasion, but, unfortunately, most of the cuts piped into my headphones came from her jazz period. Wherever she had been when she recorded these songs, whatever she hoped to accomplish, they weren't a serenade for a cancer patient in ill-fitting pajamas, a hockey mask strapped to his face, his back uncomfortably roosted on two pillows while an insane machine spun and bonged in order to take a picture of his brain.

"Brian?" I asked aloud. "Brian, can you hear me?"

He couldn't. Or he didn't. I tried to put my mind elsewhere, which is a trick I can sometimes perform. Especially at night when I had trouble sleeping, I could re-fish streams. As fuzzy as I might be about some incidents in my life, I could recall with great lucidity various streams I had fished. Lately I had been using a trip to Idaho and Montana where I had fished both the St. Joe River and the various tributaries around Kelly Creek. I had also fished a length of the legendary Blackfoot River, Norman Maclean's home water in his *A River Runs Through It*. On one particular day, when I was not at all sure if I had landed on the right section of the famous river — it's difficult to arrive as an outsider and know where to fish on any river — I had cast a Muddler Minnow down a braided stretch of white water before, suddenly, a good rainbow hit. From there I worked down the stream, perhaps the greatest hour of fishing in my life, and topped off the evening with a slow, lazy drifting fly passing beside a submerged aspen when an enormous trout rose and took my line so hard the water hissed.

"Brian, could you please turn the music off?" I asked him when I slid out halfway through the procedure so that he could put a contrast dye in my arm port.

"Do you want something else?"

"No, thanks. I'll be better off with just . . ."

"Okay," he said. "You could have used the rubber ball."

"It's fine," I said. "I'm fine."

For the rest of the session, I alternated between the wonderful mountains of Montana and the great clanging and buzzing of the MRI machine. When it finally concluded, Brian removed the port and taped me up. He gave me his hand to sit up. When I stood, my pajamas nearly shimmied off my body.

Susan met me in the waiting room.

"Are you okay?" she asked, her face tight with worry.

"I'm fine, why?"

"You were in there so long, I got nervous. I thought for sure they had discovered something, I don't know what, something that they had to record carefully . . ."

"No, it was just a long treatment. Or procedure."

"I looked it up finally and saw that it could be ninety minutes. Then I was better."

But she clearly had not been better. She pulled her bag and computer together, then we walked to the snack bar. We held hands. I told her a little of my Joni Mitchell adventure and she smiled, but, I realized, she had gone through something as I lay on the MRI rack. While I had been envisioning the bright streams of Idaho and Montana, she had been envisioning my demise, the moment when things would turn darker again.

"I come bearing good news!" Dr. Dragnev announced from the doorway of the examining room. He smiled and said hello and we greeted him in return. It was a wonderful way to start a consultation. Today, at least, the rain did not threaten to fall.

He had already previewed both the brain and chest scans. Everything, he said, remained about the same. Stability, in the cancer world, is success.

And strangely, we did not have a great deal to say as a result of the findings. In other circumstances, around a glass of wine, perhaps, we would have been chatterboxes. But this wasn't time for chitchat. We respected his expertise too much to distract from why we were there. On previous visits, we had composed a list of questions the night before, but this time we were on untested ground.

Nonetheless, there were a few surprises, mostly of the sort that arose out of something you thought you understood, but clearly didn't. While I had heard loud and clear that I should be exercising to maintain the level of fitness that I possessed, for the first time I heard Dr. Dragnev say the healthy lung tissue in both lungs might benefit from walks. That there could be a gain, in other words, an enhancement of health.

"Really?" I asked.

"Yes, of course."

That little piece of information touched me deeply. I was not, I at last understood, sick in every molecule of my body. I was still here, body and mind, and I could even prosper in a significant way. Addition was possible, not merely depletion. Then we got into a conversation — as usual — about time and conditions. Because of something he had said last time, Susan asked if he had other treatments in mind, what might be some options, what did he mean by it?

After he answered, I told him he was like the pope. We scrutinized every word.

That brought a laugh, but Susan later told me it was a courtesy laugh. We debated it on the ride home. It was the kind of thing we loved to play with, a perfect toy for our slants of mind.

We went to bed early. It had been a long day. Dr. Dragnev's final word to us had been that if I lived ten years, I would not set a record. I suspected he was being kind. As we turned off the lights and settled in, I realized that with hope came old questions. If I was going to live a decade longer, well, then all the pre-retirement questions returned. Did I keep or sell my house? Move someplace warmer, at least in the winter? Get a job of some sort, or decide to volunteer again? That was life, of course. I lay beside Susan and went through thoughts that led me to the future, a river I couldn't wait to fish.

In the interval between our visit with Dr. Dragnev and our trip to see the sandhill cranes in Nebraska, I began watching a YouTube channel hosted by a young man in Georgia whose hobby it was to lift sheets of tin that had been abandoned on the ground in order to see what snakes had collected there. Down in the notes beneath the video someone scolded him for using his bare hand, and for lifting the tin so that the opening was toward him. The scolder noted that some snakes strike immediately when they see daylight in such conditions, thinking a predator has come to devour them, and that he should pry the tins up with the opening away from him.

I found the whole concept fascinating. The young man was a "herper" who loved snakes, and he spoke with genuine passion about a coral snake — venomous — he had discovered under a plastic Tupperware lid. The tented heat, apparently, drew the snakes, where they could bake in peace and burn off the lactic acid that inhibited their vitality.

I didn't have to work hard to figure out why the search for living creatures under hot tin sheets captured my attention. A poisonous surprise? A psychological tease about what we would discover the next time we lifted my personal tin? It was too easy to deconstruct.

My first wife, Amy, wrote a short note to say that she had heard, and so forth. I wrote back and wished her well. It struck me that she wrote to me at my old work address. She didn't even know where or how I do most of my personal correspondence. Then again, I didn't know her address either. *It may be the case that this is goodbye*, I wrote at the end. She didn't reply.

Baseball resolved its labor dispute and returned to playing a game that I loved and a game that meant spring for me. My sister Cathy wrote to say she had received a new set of hearing aids — she is seventy-seven — and could hear birdsong again for the first time in years. The news made me teary with its simple goodness.

The trip to see the cranes crept closer. The airline updated our flights and scheduled our return through Denver. It added at least four hours to our trip, but the update came with no bailout option or second choice — and certainly no apology or offer of a refund or any kind of customer service upgrade. The world — in that specific way — had grown less and less to my liking. I don't think I was merely being a cranky old man to want someone to hear my complaint. The world had been gentler to customers when I was a boy, but I didn't need cancer to know that no one wants to hear a comment like that from an old man.

A spring snowstorm struck with high winds and another four or five inches of snow, but the sun was too strong for winter to intimidate us any longer. Besides, it's a well-used adage in New Hampshire that spring snow is the poor man's fertilizer. I put the last of my birdseed in the feeder and watched it disappear with the increased light and warmth; two ravens, black and startlingly large, began coming to feast on the remaining suet. One afternoon, I tried the old lawn tractor and was amazed that it started on the first turn, and I sat for a while in the sunlight, letting the engine and my winter bones bask in the fragile warmth.

In other words, life — sweet, everyday life — began again. But, of course, that was an inaccurate way to look at things. Life had always been ongoing, always churning, always bubbling. I had been the one removed for a time, sidelined, put on the bench to watch the game rather than participate. The sports metaphor — riding the bench — was reasonably apt, because I was no longer certain, given the chance, that I had the ability, much less the drive, to reenter the game. If cancer had taken me on a journey, one that was far from over, I was now returning to find the mail piled high, the houseplants too dry, the scatter of leaves from the backyard herded into a worried clump against the porch. I wanted to straighten the house, put things in order, but for the first time in my life I felt unequal to the task.

Susan suggested I trade in my old backpack for a wheeled carry-on bag. It seemed a fussy thing to do, but I knew she had a point. On my way back from visiting her, I stopped at a Goodwill store to see what they had on hand. It turns out, not much. The store happened to be near an RV center, a place I had noticed many times. I have an old A-Liner camper, essentially a tent on wheels, and I had been thinking about trading it in for something more comfortable. On a whim I pulled in and caught the staff drinking coffee and going through a morning meeting. The store was in that uncomfortable stage between winter and summer when snowmobiles are still on the sales floor beside fancy barbecue ranges. I had to wait a few minutes before a salesman, Vinny, asked what he could do for me.

As we walked toward his office, I told him my circumstances. I told him about cancer, about Tagrisso, about how much time I might have, how serious I was about a new camper. I have no idea why I chose this moment, and this person, to hear my confession. It turns out, as we sat in his antiseptic office, Vinny could not have been kinder. His wife was currently under a doctor's care for breast cancer; he himself had had his prostate removed. What had been a somewhat ridiculous, old-guy-kicking-the-tires morning drop-in had suddenly turned into a real conversation with a complete stranger. Our tones dropped; we did not joke or make small talk. He told me his dad had died of lung cancer, so he knew a little of what I was going through. When we walked the grounds, he was attentive and slow, deliberately opening doors for me, kindly answering questions without pushing any sort of sales spiel on me. The trailers were not for me — too large, too expensive — but I left that lot feeling lifted. His kindness had come, in part, from my willingness to be vulnerable. I made a deal with myself to let more people inside, to not hide my condition from quite so many people. I had to trust the kindness of strangers, as Blanche DuBois reminds us in *A Streetcar Named Desire*, though that was not easy for me.

On a warm day around this period, I brought the porch furniture out again. It was too early, really, but I couldn't help myself.

When the temperature reached sixty-one at noon, I napped on the old glider, a book spread on my chest, the clouds bright white and lovely on the White Mountains' western ridge. *I am here now*, I told myself. *I've made it to spring.* I became slightly teary thinking about how I wanted to see more springs, but then I rebuked myself and made sure I was grateful for the time I had gained. I was still a ghost of myself, a napping, slow-moving approximation of what I had been, but the world still delighted me.

"The great thing about the dead, they make space," John Updike, one of my favorite novelists, had written in *Rabbit Is Rich*, the penultimate novel in his remarkable Rabbit series. Getting a terminal diagnosis, I realized as I reclined on the glider, transformed one into a dinner guest who stayed to drink one last brandy too many. It wasn't that people minded, really, but that one's hosts couldn't keep from being a tad impatient. They were tired and ready for bed, and the meal, after all, had been carefully prepared and served. The story needed a second act; it needed action. And while I didn't think anyone was actively pulling for my death, I understood that such a diagnosis was truly a bell peal that could not be unheard. I could imagine conversations that batted me around a bit, one person asking what she or he had heard, what news they could conjure up together, both of them wondering, inevitably, about time. And about space, I suppose. The house would turn over, so would my car and fly rods and computer. Somewhere along the line, my son would decide that his dad's things had cluttered up around here long enough, and he might hire a couple of his students to carry the old papers and files out to a dumpster. That was as it should be. I would make room for him, and for whatever children he brought to our house, just as my father had made room for me. When my dad had died, I spent several weeks in the old house cleaning it out. My brothers and sisters stopped by, all of them living in the first echoes of my dad's passing, and we cooked hamburgers and drank beer and caught up with one another. Sitting in the New Jersey heat — he had died on Bastille Day — we were, tenderly and briefly, a family as we had once been a family long days before.

# 19

*Leukemia* means "white-blood." It was first called leukemia — or leukämie — in 1847 by Dr. Rudolf Virchow, a German biologist who had observed that this cancer could be readily identified by the milky tone of the patient's blood. The color of the blood resulted from an overabundance of white cells, an imbalance that was usually fatal.

Almost precisely a century later in the aftermath of World War II, Sadako Sasaki, a Japanese girl suffering from leukemia as a result of the Hiroshima bombing, began folding one thousand origami cranes in the hope that the red-capped bird would restore her to health. She was not quite twelve. She believed in the power of the crane, or *tsuru* as it is known in her home country, because it is an ancient symbol in Japanese myth and folklore, one that signified happiness and, above all, longevity. Cranes might live a thousand years, the myths promised her. They are pictured on Japanese currency and in paintings, on vases and bas-relief plaques. Cranes typically bond for life. They dance together and recognize one another's calls.

After her death, Sadako Sasaki became a symbol of the innocent victims of war. As they say in Africa, *When elephants fight, it is the grass that suffers*. She was merely collateral damage, though that is a vile, deliberately obscuring phrase to cover the rank death of a young girl. Sadako Sasaki's example of folding a thousand cranes to give flight to one's hopes spread everywhere. In my last semester of teaching, a young woman in my class showed me cranes she had been folding for her sick father. She said it was a journey, that she had started off strong, put them aside for a while, and then gradually entered a meditative approach that soothed her. I had no idea at the time why, specifically, she bothered to fold origami birds. I thought it was an online meme, a silly busy-work that she had learned somewhere. Now, with cancer, I know a different story.

Pliny the Elder wrote that one crane in every flock is set to stand guard. The crane holds a rock in its talons, so that if the crane falls asleep on its watch, the rock will fall on the ground to wake it again. In heraldry, a crane holding a stone is an often-used symbol and it is known as *crane in its vigilance*.

We were going to see the cranes. I was a little crane crazy.

I turned this picture into my screen saver. It appears in a manuscript called the Harley Bestiary from the thirteenth century. It shows a *crane vigilant*, complete with a stone in its right foot.

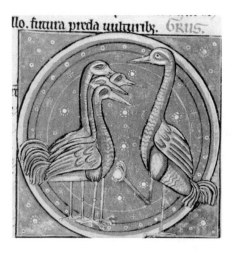

Nevertheless, as much as I thought the cranes might be something to see, something to cap off a year of living with cancer, I wasn't sure what I expected to gain by such a journey. What was driving me to make the trip? I'm not a serious birder, and neither is Susan, and though I was certain the cranes made for an interesting sight, was it worth a sort of pilgrimage to Nebraska? That was a trip of several thousands of miles; by plane it was four flights with two switchovers in Chicago, a round-trip by car to Boston, and so forth. I wondered if I wasn't setting myself up for disappointment and for the very thing I had tried not to give in to after the diagnosis: a last big act, a try at something mythic, a forced moment, in other words.

But the weather, when we scanned ahead, promised warmth. Nebraska, inviting our visit, promised March temperatures of fifty-plus. At least we had dodged the potential brutality of a late freeze. We never wavered about going, but neither did we dare predict that it would be worthwhile. We shrugged when we talked about it, one of us always adding, "It will be good to get away. Nebraska in March!"

On a Friday afternoon, we arrived at Boston's Logan airport with our binoculars packed deep inside our carry-on bags. We wore our heavy clothes and jackets. We had made a deal that this was far from a fashion show; we acknowledged we would have to wear the same thing several times. I brought an old down ski jacket and heavy walking shoes. Susan wore a gray wool watch cap and a red, boiled-wool overshirt. We looked like two people going out to ice-skate.

And so we traveled. In Chicago we had to walk from one terminal to another, a twenty-minute hike at least, and Susan wondered several times why we didn't get a *beep car*, as she called it, one with a driver that pushes its way through foot traffic in airports everywhere, to bring us to our gate. But I told her I was solid, and I was. I made the walk without difficulties, carrying my bag over my shoulder. Several times she slipped her hand onto my back to check my breathing. She didn't think I noticed, or perhaps she believed I would take it for an affectionate touch, but I appreciated her concern.

Arriving in Lincoln, Nebraska, after seven hours of travel, we rented a car and drove to a Hilton. I was tired, but not more than I might have been without cancer. We slept the night and got up early to make the two-hour drive along Route 80 to Kearney, Nebraska, in Buffalo County, where we had booked an Airbnb. Kearney, from what we had read and pieced together, was the eye of the crane hurricane. The Platte River near Kearney, which was where the cranes congregated, ran east to west through the plains, draining water to the Missouri River, then onward to the Mississippi, then finally to the Gulf of Mexico. French explorers and fur trappers used a word from the indigenous Otoe-Missouria people, calling it *Nebraskier*, which meant "flat water." From there the French phrasing, *rivière plate*, or "flat river," doubtless lent its name to the Platte River.

The landscape was flat and tireless. It's a standard joke, of course, to talk about how straight and true Route 80 is through Nebraska, but it was also factual. Fleets of semi-trucks led us down the highway, many of them pulling double freights. The fields on either side of the highway remained in their winter dormancy. It was spring by the calendar, but not by the color of the corn stubble that lay bent and broken in acre after acre. The farmers had not yet plowed, but a few had been out to clean their fields. Great wheels of hay waited like yo-yos of grass for some child-giant to come by and play with them. Here and there black Angus cattle watched from the center of an open prairie, their chins moving side-to-side to chew their perpetual cud.

We were only minutes from the Platte when Susan glanced

up, paused a second, and asked if those were cranes flying high in a lazy V. I bent down and looked through the windshield, smiled, reached for her hand, and agreed that they must be.

*At least we've seen some cranes*, I thought. As an angler, I knew how it was to go out into a river and return with nothing. Nature could give, but it could also withhold, and I thought, at that early point in our journey, that we could at least say in good conscience at our return, "Yes, we saw the cranes."

We stopped first at the Crane Trust, at the Big Bend section of the Platte River, a nonprofit conservation organization fighting to preserve the land and water needed by the cranes and other migrating birds. The weather had turned sunny and warm, and as we climbed out of our rental car, we heard the loud squawking of cranes. I'm not sure what Susan thought, but I at first imagined the Crane Trust played the sound of cranes over loudspeakers the way a haunted house on a New Jersey boardwalk might play eerie screams and ghostly boos. The sound, in other words, disappointed me by its cheesiness. But then, as we walked to the back of the Crane Trust building, we realized that the sounds were the furthest thing from artificial. Cranes — large birds roughly the size of swans — flew high in the sky over acres of meadows. Red-winged blackbirds sang their busy songs in the bushes around the building, but between notes came the steady call of the cranes, wild and haunting, that we would live with for the next few days.

Inside the Crane Trust building the docents and volunteers were elated because a whooping crane had landed in the water where a live feed held it dead center in its lens. If sandhill cranes stand around three feet tall, with a six-foot wingspan, the whooping crane is closer to five feet tall with a seven-foot wingspan, white as snow, and one of the rarest birds in the United States. It had been hunted almost to extinction — down to approximately fifteen in 1941 — for the millinery trade in the East. The feathers, in short, had been used to decorate ladies' hats, and the practice had only halted when a forward-thinking group of Connecticut women took a stand. The bird was taken for meat, too, by the early European explorers, who frequently fired indiscriminately with their harquebus shot. In 1589, Captain Amadas observed them at Wokokon Island in North Carolina, where the birds "arose, with such a crye, re-doubled by many ecchos, as if an armie of men had showted altogether."

Now that crane, white and tall and elegant, stood in midst of a flock of sandhill cranes, a lonely traveler, going north to find another of its kind, if such a one still existed. For workers and volunteers in a crane sanctuary, it was a great and important day.

A woman volunteer took out a map when we asked questions and gave us a road to take into the heart of the crane gathering. She was the best kind of volunteer — one whose joy and enthusiasm had not lessened while her knowledge had increased. Susan took on the job of navigating, which was a bit humorous because she is notoriously bad at directions. But on this trip, channeling some sort of mysterious crane power, she did not miss a turn.

We set off, heading roughly toward the Rowe Sanctuary, another crane preserve, which marked the western edge of the crane habitat. Between the two crane reserves, six hundred thousand cranes had already collected. Some, as it turned out, had recently caught a southern thermal pushing them northward on their migrations. But thousands upon thousands still waited in the spring cornfields, feeding up for the demands of their migration on the refuse corn spilled during the harvest each year.

I drove slowly. Susan kept a map open on her lap and gradually traced the turns we needed to make. I felt good. I felt alive. I was not a cancer patient in those moments; I was a slightly confused, optimistic crane enthusiast, come to witness one of the great animal migrations on earth. At this point, however, we had only seen cranes high among the clouds, beads of black against the limitless Nebraska sky. We heard them everywhere around us, but I wondered, somewhat cynically, if this event had been oversold. It's common among fishermen to hear, *You should have been here yesterday when they were really biting*, and I worried that we had — I had — misjudged the timing.

And then we found them. At first — we conferred about this afterward — I thought the birds, pewter-colored and blended into the bare soil of the cornfields, were old farm tires, set out on the ground to anchor a tarp. Susan, a New Englander to her core, thought they were stone walls. We kept looking and driving slower. Inch by inch, we began to comprehend what lay before us. What I had taken for old tires, and Susan for stone walls, turned out not to be a flock of cranes, but a sea of cranes, a vast calling sea, that stretched beyond our ability to understand. We reached for each other's hand. I felt my eyes grow damp.

They were here, after all. They were here as they had been for millions of years. They were, by many estimates, the oldest avian species left on earth. Now, once our eyes grew accustomed to what we were seeing, the cranes seemed almost unfathomable, like looking, I imagined, at a lottery ticket in your hand that held the winning numbers. You could read the numbers a hundred times, but your mind remained back a step, trying to frame what you observed, because no one could conceive of a mass of birds like the one feeding on the field on the first encounter.

"Look," Susan said, pointing and pointing, trying to under-stand that the flock did not end here, or there, but went on for a quarter mile, gray birds, massive birds, who sometimes took flight, and sometimes landed with their wings out, their legs and chests pushed forward like children hanging from the low bar of a jungle gym. Or no, like pterodactyls, ancient creatures, somehow alive today, this moment, flying without caution in the blond sunshine of a Nebraska spring.

*I can't believe what I'm seeing,* I said or she said, and our voices hardly mattered. This was beyond speech or words. The enormous urge to live, the great desire to procreate, to continue, to carry on, rested in every molecule the birds inhabited. This was why we had come. This was a rendezvous as old as any on earth, and we were a part of it, a minor part, to be sure, but a witness nevertheless. Seen from above by satellite, the birds in flight formed clouds, wind made visible, and all the beauty of the earth asked to be remembered here.

Several times, while Susan was busy scanning the birds, I had to lower my eyes to keep from weeping. I could not kid myself; this, precisely, was what cancer would take from me. The beauty that sustained me, the sunrises and sunsets, the seals blowing air in the water beyond our land in Maine, a wood thrush singing deep in the woods, a lilac, a clock ticking, all would perish when the cancer grew strong enough to defeat the drugs that protected me. I gave in to it readily, it would win eventually, but that does not mean that I would not miss this rare earth, deeply and vividly, and lament the loss of the wind on my face, the awkwardly graceful leap of a crane to pair-bond with its mate.

We looked as long as we could still absorb their beauty, and in the morning we rose in darkness and went to a public viewing platform where our volunteer from the Crane Trust had promised us good viewing. We stood with twenty or thirty others in the cold wind, our coats buttoned tight around our necks, our gloved hands trembling a little with the weight of our binoculars. In time, in silence, the sun began to show in the east, and I thought of *The Odyssey*, Homer's rosy-fingered dawn, but it was not a moment for reflection of that kind. Then the light revealed the cranes. They stood in water — water protects them by sounding an alarm if a predator begins to splash toward them during the night — and the sunlight gave them shadows. The shadows rippled on the surface of the water, and the cranes, hungry now, restless, began to move and dance and prod. I kept my binoculars to my eyes for fear I would cave in if I gave in to the emotion that roared inside me. Cancer had not won or lost; such thinking was ridiculous. Cancer simply existed, part of it all, a shadow on the water, rippling, waiting to be made full by the sun.

And then the birds rose up. They *kettled*, as the biologists call it. Ten thousand birds, twenty thousand up and down the river, who could say? I felt my heart lift and fill, and I rose with them. They made a heavenly racket. I flew north on the warm thermals, a trip of five thousand miles ahead of us, and the land beneath me spun past like a log turning slowly in a northern river. I held out my hand to Susan and she took it, keeping me here a little longer, her own flight years away, but mine, as we both understood, waited for the instant our fingers would part, the wind inevitable and not a thing to fear.

# Acknowledgments

John Updike, one of my favorite authors, once wrote that he hoped his novels would be discovered someday on a library shelf by a young woman or man, the book jacket removed, all reviews and comments erased so that the story, and the young reader, would meet as all authors hope their works are met: honestly and without fanfare, one human speaking, across miles and ages, to another. The writing of this short book sustained me during a difficult time, and it's my hope that I fairly represent one person's experience with cancer. I dedicated this book to my fellow cancer patients at the outset, and I repeat that dedication here. I wish you all well. I wish grace and dignity for you. I hope you are surrounded by love and kindness and that you don't forget to look up, when you are able, to see the birds and the sky.

But we are here now! This instant, this hour! So why the hell not? I want to thank everyone in the world! I want to thank the drivers who never veered across the roadway to kill me, the sharks that didn't eat me, the psychopaths who left me alone. Thanks to the diner cooks who prepared my pancakes, to the mechanics who worked on my vehicles, to the Africans who taught me kindness, to the plumbers who rigged up my hot water and septic system, to the woodcutters who brought me oak and maple and birch. To my coaches, to my colleagues, to my teammates, to my opponents, to anyone and everyone who gave my small boat a shove down stream, thank you. Thank you to the trees and rivers and trout who turned me inside out. Thanks to all the dogs I've loved, those sweet, sweet open hearts whose goodness never failed. Thanks to a few cats, too, and to the manufacturers of Cheerios, my childhood breakfast. Special appreciation to the farmers who grew summer tomatoes and ears of corn that held the salt and the evening's coolness in their flesh. It was all pretty wonderful when I think about it.

On a more practical level, I want to express my thanks to all those near to me who helped with this book. Susan, of course, before everything. She read every word and talked to me about my meaning in our wonderful Morning Show. 6, Susan, always and forever, 6.

Thanks also to my son, Justin, who made me laugh and fed me Party-for-Two cakes and always treated me with love and tenderness. To Chip Fleischer, my editor and friend; my agents, Christina and Andrea; and all others at Steerforth who brought this book to print, thank you. I suspect you can guess how much this work meant to me, and you made it possible.

Thanks, also, to Maria Popova, writer and editor of *Marginalia*, whose brilliant blog and newsletter often fed me with what she calls *timeless nourishment*. I read her quotes and curated pieces with deep pleasure and frequently bounced off one or two in the composition of this book.

To the doctors and staff at Dartmouth-Hitchcock, thank you. The work you do on behalf of your countless patients is beyond calculation. You gave me time, and who in this world can give more?

And lastly, thanks to the cranes of Nebraska who come and go each season. Good winds to you.